M000287011

Diagnosing and Treating Addictions

An Integrated Approach to Substance Use Disorders and Concurrent Disorders

by
DR. MERVILLE VINCENT

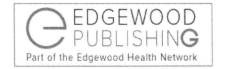

Edgewood Publishing • Toronto, Canada

Edgewood Publishing
Edgewood Health Network, Inc.
39 Pleasant Boulevard
Toronto, ON M4T 1K2, Canada

Library and Archives Canada Cataloguing in Publication

Vincent, Merville, author
Diagnosing and treating addictions : An integrated approach to substance use disorders and concurrent disorders / by Dr. Merville Vincent.

Includes bibliographical references.
ISBN-13: 978-0-9937409-1-6 (pbk.) (Edgewood Treatment Center)
ISBN-10: 099374091X

1. Dual diagnosis. 2. Dual diagnosis – Treatment. 3. Substance abuse – Diagnosis. 4. Substance abuse – Treatment. I. Title.

RC564.68.V55 2014   616.86   C2014-905780-6

Contents

Tables

Preface

Life has a way of catching you in its current and taking you along a stream that you would have least anticipated. Coincidence? Fate? Higher power? We get pushed along, working hard "one day at a time," and after enough time, major changes unfold!

One of those streams is the path of my training and experience that led to my current position in addiction medicine and addiction psychiatry. I completed a bachelor of applied science degree in human nutrition from the University of Guelph in 1980 and a master's degree, also in nutrition, from the University of Toronto in 1983 (completed during medical school). After that, I went to the McMaster school of medicine, where I graduated in 1984. My psychiatry residency followed.

Then, in 1988, I took on a position as a general psychiatrist on one of the general psychiatry units at the Homewood Health Centre in Guelph, Ontario. I felt confident and comfortable in this new position, and worked with a team of health professionals who took pride in their work and had compassion for their patients.

A particular concern lingered. This very large hospital, with over 300 patients, also had a specialized addiction treatment unit with over sixty beds. Patients were routinely admitted for both detoxification and ongoing treatment of their addiction. At that time, treatment was primarily a twenty-eight-day program. When I was on call after hours, I would frequently receive calls from the nursing staff requesting advice or orders for patients undergoing withdrawal or with very specific addiction issues. I became acutely aware that my medical training and subsequent psychiatric training had not prepared me to address addiction issues competently. I do recall discussion of various medical illnesses that were caused by addiction; however, detoxification and general treatment for addiction had not been an area of teaching or study. It became evident that this was not simply a deficiency in my personal training, or my university, but was a problem of much greater magnitude generally in medicine and psychiatry.

After two years of doing general psychiatry, and increasingly feeling a need to develop more expertise in the area of addiction medicine, I approached the medical director of the addiction program with a request to spend three months working in the addiction program, where I would be able to learn about addictions and provide psychiatric consultation to addiction patients at the hospital. The director gladly accommodated this request, as the centre did not have any ongoing psychiatrist on the service and it would clearly be a mutually beneficial arrangement. I was very excited about this transition, although I also felt somewhat inadequate. My last three years at Homewood were a full-time addiction practice.

I was immediately struck by several major differences between the general psychiatry program and the addiction program. Most strikingly, all the other physicians working in the addiction program were in their own recovery from addictions. This was not unusual at that time — most physicians working in the area of addiction medicine had developed an interest through their own recovery. They were able to relate very well to many of the patients through their own struggle with addiction and recovery — but I was the odd man out. I was somewhat of a misfit because, in many ways my personal background could not of made for a worse fit. I felt somewhat handicapped in my work. Both of my grandfathers had been Baptist ministers, and both were vehemently opposed to use of alcohol, which they regarded as a sin. My paternal grandfather had been actively involved in the prohibition movement and, to my knowledge, had never had a drink. My father, a physician, certified in internal medicine and psychiatry, was a very active member of the Baptist community, and to my knowledge was also a complete abstainer from alcohol. He had always received a special insurance rate for his car insurance on the basis of his being an abstainer from alcohol!

However, as it turned out, my genetic makeup was in the area of addiction medicine and addiction psychiatry, rather than as a patient suffering with addiction. My father developed an expertise in the area of addiction psychiatry decades before I began working in the field, and was recognized as an expert in the area of addicted health professionals, and in particular, the women who were increasingly entering the field of medicine.

I felt extremely naïve and inexperienced working with this population of patients. I had never used marijuana or street drugs. After a couple of drunken episodes on a school trip age of eighteen, I had also chosen to only drink socially. I generally did not like the feeling of being intoxicated and I certainly did not like the feeling of being hung over! The advantage that I did have was having a much better sense of "healthy," in terms of relationship and behaviours, than many of them had had the opportunity to learn.

I was also struck by the significant difference in language and the means of understanding problems and behaviours. Spirituality was not a particularly valued area of study in psychiatry at that time. I had never learned about the twelve steps and certainly had never heard of *thirteen-stepping* (Alcoholics Anonymous slang for getting into relationships with others in the program); *dry drunk* and *postacute withdrawal* had never been a part of my lexicon.

Sponsors and temporary sponsors had never been a part of my life. *Codependency* and *adult children of alcoholics* were new terms for me. I had not really thought about addiction as a disease.

I was also unfamiliar with the medicine of addictions. I had no familiarity with *front-end loads* (see chapter 7) and had never prescribed medications such as methadone, Antabuse, or Temposil. I had very limited experience helping people detoxify from alcohol and benzodiazepines, and no experience at all helping people detoxify from opiates.

The beauty of doing something new and unfamiliar is that you are working on the steep part of the learning curve! At the end of three months, I found that I loved working with alcoholics and drug addicts. I marvelled at the dramatic change in their lives over a period of four weeks. People walked out of treatment looking dramatically improved with a solid plan for recovery that would lead to success if they followed the aftercare recommendations that were given to them. I was also struck by the apparent difference in focus of responsibility for wellness. In some ways, a large part of psychiatric treatment felt like the physician's responsibility to select and administer the right medications for the best result. Patients obviously had some responsibility for their own wellness as well, but addiction recovery was clearly placed in the hands of the recovering person, who was expected to follow up on wellness behaviours in order to get well.

The three-year period at Homewood was highly rewarding. The area of concurrent disorders— treating patients with addiction problems as well as an identified psychiatric disorder—was developing and I became quite involved in teaching in this area. I appreciated the mentorship I had received during this time, particularly from the physician who was the director of the program, and also from many others who patiently guided and educated me through this experience.

I successfully passed the American Society of Addiction Medicine examination in 1992. I reluctantly left my position as addiction psychiatrist after being tempted by a position as a rural psychiatrist on Vancouver Island, and moved there in 1993 with my family, where I again practised general psychiatry for the next decade. One-third of my practice was spent in the inpatient psychiatry unit, another third providing office consultations for family physicians, and another third working in a mental health clinic with patients with serious and persistent mental illness, primarily psychosis and mood disorders.

Obviously addiction medicine was now a component of any medical practice, and I saw my fair share of patients with addiction disorders. My previous training in addiction was an invaluable tool in all the clinical settings. After a decade of working in this community, I became interested in an excellent residential program nearby, called Edgewood. This 120-bed addiction treatment facility had opened up some years previously and had continually expanded. Edgewood provides withdrawal services and residential treatment for a wide range of addiction disorders. It had strong links with the forestry industry, where a need for residential addiction treatment in British Columbia had grown. The timing for my contact was perfect, as they had recently lost their last psychiatrist and were actively seeking another addiction psychiatrist. Within a short period of time, I was working full-time in this program and I have been there for the last twelve years, as the director of psychiatric services.

In the last two years I became a certificant of the Canadian Society of Addiction Medicine and completed the Medical Review Officer certification examination in the area of occupational addiction medicine and drug testing. Additionally, I served as the president of the British Columbia Psychiatric Association for two years, following which I was the addiction medicine representative for this organization.

I am currently a clinical instructor in the addiction division of the Department of Psychiatry at University of British Columbia, where we routinely provide supervision of medical students and residents in their training to become psychiatrists and family physicians. We have had addiction medicine/addiction psychiatry elective students from across Canada and occasionally internationally.

In addition to on-site addiction training, I've had the opportunity to do considerable teaching in the area of addiction medicine and psychiatry as an invited speaker at hospital rounds and at a variety of conferences. I was particularly delighted to be able to present rounds at St. Paul's Hospital in Vancouver, with my psychiatrist father as copresenter, on the subject of addiction in health care professionals. I have presented many talks in the area of concurrent disorders including PTSD (posttraumatic stress disorder) and addiction, mood disorders and addiction, psychosis and addiction, detoxification, addiction in health professionals, methamphetamine, and occupational addiction medicine.

I am the codirector of the physician training program at Edgewood, providing addiction training for community physicians, primarily in the area of psychiatry and family practice, although we have had clinical leaders in other fields participate as well. This program has been accredited for twenty-eight hours of continuing medical education credits. We have had over 100 participants through this program since its inception, with glowing reviews.

I have been fortunate to spend the last twelve years in this rich environment!

Chapter 1

Introduction

I vividly recall visiting a remote hospital in an impoverished area of South Africa at the age of 18. My physician father had been invited to give a series of lectures to medical staff there. The hospital was situated on top of a hill. Patients were on blankets on the floor, surrounded by a couple of family members. The facilities were extremely sparse and limited.

It was approaching dusk when we began to hear singing from the village down below. It was a Friday night. Absolutely beautiful music drifted up to our perch on the hill, and we could imagine that the singing and dancing at this community gathering was a time of celebration, and escape, from the hardship of day-to-day life. We soon learned that the villagers were drinking a fermented alcoholic beverage, no doubt very different from the type we were used to seeing in North America.

Alcohol, in particular, has been widely available in many countries of the world for thousands of years. Similarly, drugs in various forms have also clearly played different roles, and served different functions in society. Opium — sometimes called the "joy plant" — has been used for both medicinal and other purposes in many countries of the world, and has been cultivated since at least 3400 BCE. We know that the opium trade was active in 1300 BCE and that opium has been in almost continuously high demand for both medicinal and recreational purposes. In other regions, the coca plant, marijuana, peyote, and many other natural substances have been used for the purpose of intoxication and spiritual or religious rituals.

If we consider more modern times, alcohol and drug use have been through a number of significant evolutions. The distillation process allowed for much more concentrated forms of alcoholic beverage. Morphine, a much more potent opiate, was isolated from opium in 1804. It was subsequently introduced commercially in 1827 and the hypodermic syringe was available by 1853. This led to a dramatic escalation in addiction to opiates, as well as to an intramuscular delivery system. By 1874, heroin was synthesized, and heroin use reached epidemic proportions by the early 1900s ("Opium Throughout History" 2014). Increasingly, physicians used opiates for a variety of conditions, for pain management in particular. Addiction issues became problematic.

Addiction medicine began to evolve into a specialty of its own. The *Journal of Inebriety* was started in 1876, to enhance the study of "inebriates." A number of private and public facilities became available for the treatment of alcoholics (as they are now called) and opiate addicts, many of whom would have been addicted to prescription opiates at that time. Well-documented societal struggles took place in terms of understanding addiction. A number of specialist physicians adopted a disease concept of addiction, although this was certainly not the predominant theme of the time. According to a review by William White (2012), the *Journal of Inebriety* noted more than thirty-eight intoxicating agents in its major and minor articles: "Alcohol, opiates and tobacco dominated the subject matter, accounting for 88% of the major and minor articles that focused on a particular intoxicating agent. The rank ordering of these substances was alcohol 57%, opiates 21%, tobacco 9%, coca and cocaine 5%."

While addiction to intoxicating substances is far from a new problem, significant changes in the modern era have led to even more challenges. Chemistry has advanced considerably, leading to isolation and synthesis of many new compounds. Alcohol and cigarettes are widely and easily available in spite of the known medical consequences of their use. According to the most recent World Health Organization statistics:

The harmful use of alcohol is a component cause of more than 200 disease and injury conditions in individuals, most notably alcohol dependence, liver cirrhosis, cancers and injuries. In 2012, about 3.3 million net deaths, or 5.9 percent of all global deaths, were attributable to alcohol consumption. In 2012, 139 million net disability-adjusted life years, or 5.1 percent of the global burden of disease and injury, were attributable to alcohol consumption. At least 15.3 million persons have drug use disorders. (World Health Organization 2012)

The National Institute of Drug Abuse provides a similarly sobering account: "abuse of tobacco, alcohol and illicit drugs cost over $600 billion annually in costs related to crime, lost work productivity and health care. Health care costs alone attributable to tobacco are $96 billion, alcohol $30 billion, and illicit drugs $11 billion" (National Institute on Drug Abuse 2013).

Gaming addiction is increasing. In these addictions, adolescents and adults compulsively spend hours a day playing video games on their computers or gaming machines, with associated negative consequences.

Technology developments have also been a significant factor in the dramatic escalation in behavioural addictions. Consider its impact on gambling. In Canada alone, total revenue generated from government operated gaming was almost $14 billion, with highest revenues in Ontario. The National Council on Problem Gambling estimates that two million Americans, or about 1 percent of the population, are pathological gamblers. An additional 2 to 3 percent, or four to six million people, would be considered problem gamblers — people whose gambling affects their everyday lives.

Technology has also made its impact on sexually addictive behaviours. Pornography has never been more easily available than in recent years. Social media has provided an additional mechanism for facilitating affairs and subsequent marital disruption. Specialized websites allow escorts to advertise their services, and partners who wish to cheat on their husbands and wives can do so, courtesy of sites specializing in this purpose.

Even though addiction has been with us for centuries, recent changes are having a significantly negative impact on many individuals, families, and our society at large. For this reason, it is essential that we develop a further understanding of addiction and implement various means to address this problem.

In addition to my personal baseline interest in teaching general principles of addiction to various health professionals, I felt it was time to write this book because of several significant recent developments in the field that have surfaced in the last year. Key assessment and treatment tools have changed. The American Psychiatric Association's *Diagnostic and Statistical Manual of Mental Disorders,* known as the *DSM*, was updated to a fifth edition in May 2013. It contains a number of changes in the diagnostic criteria and description of various psychiatric disorders, including substance use disorders.

The *American Society of Addiction Medicine Patient Placement Criteria – 2 Revised*, known as the *PPC-2R*, was also recently revised and retitled; its new title is the *ASAM Criteria*. The revision incorporates a number of significant changes that relate to matching patients who have a range of severity of addiction disorders to appropriate treatment settings.

There has been considerable interest in the legalizing of marijuana, leading to significant changes in the administration of medical marijuana programs in both Canada and the United States.

We have all been affected by news of dramatic escalations in accidental deaths caused by opiate overdoses.

Lastly, major corporations and employers have been profoundly impacted by addiction and mental health issues in the workplace. As a result, employers have begun focusing attention on identifying and managing addiction disorders. Several high-profile legal cases particularly related to employers' attempts to incorporate drug screening protocols have been the result.

My goal was to write a book that would be useful for various health professionals, but expressed in language that would also make it accessible to individuals and families who may wish to learn more about addiction. Most health professionals recognize that their training is inadequate in the area of addictions. I have been told this repeatedly by medical students and residents, as well as over 100 physicians who have attended our physician training program in addiction at Edgewood. I am also aware that consumers of addiction treatment are often sophisticated and well educated, as a result of their own reading and access to resources online.

It is with great humility that I offer this book, to highlight what I feel are important practical areas, both old and new, in the wide-ranging field of addiction.

Chapter 2

What Causes Addiction?

People are baffled by addiction. Friends and families of addiction patients inevitably ask: What causes addiction? Patients will ask: Why do I do this?

Speaking from his decades in the field of addiction medicine, Dr. George Vaillant (2003) looks at addiction in terms of risk factors. He breaks these usefully into three: the agent, the environment, and the host (see table 1).

Table 1
Risk Factors for Addiction

Agent (substance)	Environment	Host
Availability	Occupation	Genetic predisposition
Cost	Peer group	Multiproblem family
Rapidity with which the agent reaches the brain	Culture	Comorbid psychiatric disorder
Efficacy of the agent as a tranquilizer	Social stability	

Availability

A substance's availability is influenced by a number of factors, many of which are dictated at a societal level. Some substances (food, alcohol) are legally available, some are illegal (cocaine, heroin), and some, chiefly marijuana, lie somewhere in between. One sees the effects of availability in clinical practice in many ways. Many individuals first use cocaine while they are drinking at a bar, club, or party where cocaine happens to be available; they had not previously considered using cocaine until the availability was there. Another common pattern involves changing availability associated with relationships. In my practice, several patients' drug of choice might fluctuate depending on who they are in a relationship with, and their partner's drug of choice. Recently, a patient of mine described how his addiction to cocaine escalated when he moved in with a roommate who was a cocaine dealer.

A recent phenomenon involving availability was Health Canada's 2012 removal from the market of the very popular—and extensively abused—prescription opiate, OxyContin. They decided to replace it with an alternative, OxyNEO, that would be less subject to abuse. Some opiate-dependent individuals then switched to heroin and a so-called "street OxyContin" began to appear. This version of the drug contains fentanyl, which is much more potent and has led to numerous accidental overdoses. Ketamine, a veterinary anesthetic agent, has also recently become much more widely available from illicit sources.

At one time, a middle-aged, male alcoholic with no history of street drug use was in our program at Edgewood. After completing residential treatment he returned home, where he began to attend regular Alcoholics Anonymous (AA) meetings. He met a woman at those meetings who was primarily addicted to cocaine. They started a relationship, and she relapsed to cocaine. She offered him cocaine repeatedly, which he consistently declined until one time, during sexual activity, she inhaled crack cocaine and blew it into his mouth, at which time he experienced a high. They did this several times until he eventually became addicted to crack cocaine as well.

Genetic Factors

The role of genetic factors in the development of substance use disorders — particularly alcohol dependence — has been widely studied. Research in this field has progressed rapidly (National Institutes of Health, 2012). Initial evidence showed that the risk of developing alcohol dependence was higher in monozygotic twins as opposed to fraternal twins; genetically vulnerable children, adopted at infancy to nonalcoholic families, retained their risk of becoming alcoholic. However, at this time, there is no specific single gene known to cause alcohol dependence or drug addiction. Substance use disorders are clearly complex and involve a number of biological factors, implying the involvement of several genes. Nevertheless, current estimates are that 50 to 60 percent of the risk of alcoholism is due to genetics.

More recently, an added focus has been placed on something called *epigenetics*. Explained simply, human beings have forty-six chromosomes, consisting of twenty-two pairs of autosomes and one pair of sex chromosomes. One member of each pair of chromosomes comes from the mother's egg cells and the other comes from the father's sperm cells. These chromosomes, organized in long chains of DNA, are tightly wound around proteins called *histone proteins*, which provide support and play a role in the activity of the genes. The human *genome* encompasses the complete set of genetic material that determines the development of an organism and all its traits and characteristics. In comparison, in the human *epigenome,* chemical modifications occur within a genome without changing the DNA sequence. Epigenetic alterations may include the direct addition of methyl groups and the chemical modification of the proteins around which the DNA is wrapped to form the chromosomes. Both of these mechanisms work in concert to remodel the structure of the protein-DNA complex, regulating the genes' expression.

What does all this contribute to the discussion of addiction? Quite a lot, according to a group of authors from Houston:

These epigenetic factors may alter initial response to a drug, continued response, the development of tolerance leading to addiction, as well as withdrawal and relapse. Emotional stressors and social adversities may cause an initial epigenetic response that alters reward-signaling pathways, predisposing one to a positive response to drug use. With chronic drug abuse and development of addiction, other epigenetic changes may occur that oppose the initial acute drug response, as illustrated by c-fos activity and cocaine in the nucleus accumbens. From the studies presented above, it appears that epigenetic changes found to be in association with drug addiction are primarily indicative of an epigenetic response to substance exposure, rather than a biological predisposition to develop an addiction. However, studies on the DNA methylation changes found in drug addiction suggest a possible role for epigenetics in predisposing an individual to an increased vulnerability for addiction. (Nielsen et al., 2012)

What this means is that, through epigenetic activity, early childhood events or traumas can alter which genes are activated, even though the genes themselves remain the same. The activation of these genes can impact vulnerability to addiction or other mental health problems. Importantly, the activated state of these genes can in turn be inherited by the next generation, in a process known as epigenetic inheritance. This is at least one mechanism that bridges our early childhood experience or adversity and the subsequent risk of developing addiction.

The Reward System

The most prominent understanding of addiction in the modern era is that addiction is a disease involving dysregulation of the brain's reward pathway. It has long been established that if you place an electrode in specific regions of a laboratory animal's brain, and the animal is able to press a lever to stimulate this area, it will do so to the exclusion of food, drinking, and other natural reward behaviours. This now well-established reward pathway involves connections between various areas of the brain — the ventral tegmental area, the nucleus accumbens, and the prefrontal cortex — comprising a region of the brain that is very important for reinforcing behaviours that promote adaptation as a species. These include sexual, eating, social, and other functions that are experienced as pleasurable. The reward system is mediated by dopamine, a neurochemical that mediates pleasurable experience. When substances of abuse are taken, they activate the reward system in a way that significantly exceeds normal pleasurable experiences.

Cocaine, crack cocaine, and methamphetamine act directly on dopamine, thus providing an excellent illustration of the changes that take place in the reward pathway with continued use. The initial use of cocaine or methamphetamine causes a dramatic elevation of dopamine in the reward pathway, generally translating into a highly positive or pleasurable experience. Almost without exception, addicts in my practice report that their first use of cocaine is highly memorable. Most will state that they felt powerful, euphoric, and highly stimulated. On a few occasions, some have even described it as "what has been missing in my life." But as these drug users continue to use, they note that it becomes harder to get the same high that they experienced at first. This is particularly true when the use is repeated and regular.

The reason is that human physiology works to maintain a stable equilibrium in various systems, including the reward system. Compare this to going on a diet: at first, weight loss is relatively easy, but it becomes progressively more difficult as the person continues to diet. The body recognizes the drop in calories, and responds to the caloric deprivation, adapting its metabolic machinery to recalibrate the body's use of carbohydrates, proteins, and fats. Similarly, with repeated use of drugs, the brain responds by trying to minimize the impact of these dopamine surges in an attempt to maintain equilibrium, in a process is called *neuroadaptation*. In an attempt to reduce the impact of elevated dopamine, the body changes the number and quality of brain receptors where dopamine exerts its action, reducing its impact. This leads to *tolerance,* where more substance is needed to generate the same effect. So the addict will start to take more and more of the substance in order to achieve the same high.

This process is important in understanding why addicts escalate their substance use. It is also very important in understanding what happens when addicts suddenly stop using their substance of choice — the brain goes into a down-regulated state, in which time must elapse before the body can return to its previous equilibrium. An interesting opposing process also occurs. When tolerance develops, it becomes harder and harder to get high, and the opposite is also true when addicts suddenly stop using: cravings for the substance become stronger and stronger. This biological process is referred to as *sensitization* or *kindling.* As we will see later, sensitization also appears to come into play in cocaine-, crack cocaine-, or methamphetamine-induced psychosis or paranoia. Once an addict begins to experience psychotic symptoms as part of the high, this particular pathway becomes sensitized and it becomes an increasingly normal part of getting high.

As addicts continue to repeatedly use cocaine, crack cocaine, and methamphetamine, they begin to develop associations with the people and places they use with. This then creates very strong triggers or cues, which remind the brain about using and getting high. Research tells us that people begin to experience dopamine elevation and a form of high before even touching the drug, simply from the anticipation of reward or using. This is why twelve-step programs and cognitive behavioural treatments speak about avoiding "slippery people and places" as a core part of recovery behaviour.

The strength of the reward pathway also increases when drug use continues, and increasingly dictates decision-making and behaviour. Located in what has often been called the reptilian brain because of its association with survival, the reward pathway operates very instinctively and very rapidly. The reward "brain" competes with the judgment "brain" for ultimate choice of behaviour. The problem is, the judgment brain is much slower to act than the reward brain. In a process that neurobiologists call salience attribution, different decision-making choices have a different value at different times, depending on whether the brain is in reward mode or judgment mode. A battle develops between the two modes, which people see when dealing with a loved one or patient. When a patient is in reward mode, there is only one thing that is important—acquiring the substance of choice and feeding the reward brain.

Addicts in early recovery may engage in various mood altering behaviours, presumably as a replacement for the alcohol and drug use that they have left behind, and the associated stimulation of reward pathways. One of the ways this may manifest in residential treatment is with flirtation and sexual relationships with other patients. In many residential treatment programs, this is looked at as relapse, and patients can be discharged for these behaviours. (See chapter 10 for a discussion of twelve-step facilitation therapy in residential treatment and for a discussion of relapse.)

In my clinical work, I repeatedly meet highly intelligent, productive, and educated people who suffer from addiction. By the time they come to Edgewood, they have typically lost all of the things that they have valued in their life: their marriages, relationships with their children, and their jobs; they have suffered financial ruin, destruction of their physical health, and legal charges; all in their pursuit of activating the reward centre of their brain.

On top of the self-destruction and decay that happens to one's sense of self, a highly painful aspect of addiction is how it hurts the very people who are most loved. Some of the most distressed people I see in my practice are mothers, in treatment for addiction, who know that they have neglected or in other ways harmed their own children. They are devastated to be away from their family for the two months of their treatment, but they know that if they don't get treatment, the destruction will continue.

In the end, the best way of understanding addiction may be that the reward brain is holding the judgment brain hostage. Unless the reward system can be suppressed, and the judgment brain enhanced and strengthened, the process will continue to progressively wreak havoc. To cope with the devastation of this process, addicts must continuously deny their reality. One of the most challenging problems in treatment is that people continue to trust their own judgment and decision-making, in spite of the obvious fact that their own best thinking has brought them to where they now are. Simply stopping the substance use or the addictive behaviour through detoxifying, or being in the early stages of treatment, does not and cannot suddenly undo processes that have taken months or years to develop. The reward brain/judgment brain battle continues to be active, even in the absence of the addictive substance or behaviour. The little red devil on the left shoulder hands out advice and the distorted perspective that aims to protect the disease, allowing it to continue, while the white angel on the right shoulder gives an entirely different opinion. The treatment process becomes a battleground.

Chapter 3

Pharmacology

In this chapter, I'll take a moment to review some important concepts and then look at specific substances.

Substance use disorders are created when various substances are repeatedly taken into the body. Substances come in a variety of forms. Some, most notably alcohol, are liquid. Others substances come in pill form. Common examples include many prescription medications such as the narcotic painkillers, and benzodiazepines such as Valium or Ativan. Some illicit drugs, such as Ecstasy or MDMA, also come in pill form. Cocaine is sold as a powder, and crack cocaine and crystal methamphetamine are available in crystalline, smokable form. Various drugs can be dissolved in liquid and then injected.

The objective for the user is to have the active substance absorbed into the body—notably, into the brain—for the purposes of getting high. Most substances will also affect other organs of the body, causing a variety of effects in addition to the desired high. Typically, drugs enter the body when they are swallowed, snorted up through the nose, smoked, or injected.

Generally speaking, substances that are swallowed have a slower onset of action. Tablets or liquids need to enter the gastrointestinal system and be absorbed into the bloodstream before they are able to reach the brain. Often, users crush and snort pills so that they can experience the high more rapidly. Smoking tobacco, crack cocaine, or heroin also allows users to experience a speedier high, since lungs have a very rich blood supply and rapid circulation to the brain. This is also the case when drugs are injected; they enter the bloodstream directly, and the active drug is taken to the brain. A very rapid onset of action is highly reinforcing.

In addition to euphoria, which is the desired effect, substances have various other effects. Some drugs, described on the street as *downers*, generally have a more calming action, although an initial burst of energy may be experienced before the sedative effect kicks in. Typical examples include opiates such as various painkillers, as well as heroin, alcohol, marijuana, and benzodiazepines and various other sedatives. GHB is a drug that behaves very much like alcohol and is preferred by some over alcohol as it is less likely to cause hangovers.

On the other hand, some drugs, described on the street as *uppers*, are well-known stimulants. Common examples include cocaine, crack cocaine, and methamphetamine, which are all street drugs. Addicts generally make a point of differentiating between cocaine and crack cocaine, even though they differ only in the route of administration. They both contain cocaine as an active ingredient. Addicts and clinicians generally look at crack cocaine addiction as a more serious drug addiction, a sign of further progression of the addiction disorder.

Some pharmaceutical stimulants, including various formulations of Dexedrine and Ritalin, are also abused and have a street value. MDMA and Ecstasy also tend to behave as stimulants. Other less common stimulants include "bath salts," which have garnered significant attention in the media lately, and PCP (also known as angel dust). In addition to euphoria, stimulants tend to cause elevations in body temperature, heart rate, and blood pressure. They may also lead to dehydration. The side effects can be extremely dangerous and may lead to acute heart problems, seizures, and death.

Nicotine

Tobacco use is the leading preventable cause of disease, disability, and death in the United States. According to the Centers for Disease Control and Prevention, cigarette smoking results in more than 443,000 premature deaths in the United States each year—about one in every five U.S. deaths, and an additional 8.6 million people suffer a serious illness caused by smoking (National Institute on Drug Abuse 2012). Nicotine is available in several forms including cigars, pipe tobacco, snuff, and chewing tobacco. Nicotine stimulates the adrenal glands, releasing the hormone epinephrine, which causes increased blood pressure, respiratory rate, and heart rate. Additionally, nicotine increases dopamine in the reward areas of brain, through the activation of nicotinic acetylcholine receptors, accounting for its addictive nature (National Institute on Drug Abuse 2012). Burning tobacco produces seven thousand different compounds, at least sixty-nine of which have been shown to be carcinogenic, and many others are known toxins (Potts and Daniels 2014). Individuals who quit smoking prior to the age of fifty reduce by half the risk of dying in the next fifteen years.

A more recent trend in cigarette smoking involves the use of electronic cigarettes:

Electronic cigarettes, often called e-cigarettes, are battery-operated devices designed to look like regular tobacco cigarettes. Like their conventional counterparts, electronic cigarettes contain nicotine. An atomizer heats a liquid containing nicotine, turning it into a vapor that can be inhaled and creating a vapor cloud that resembles cigarette smoke. The Food and Drug

Administration has questioned the safety of these products. A warning was subsequently released. (Dale 2014)

E-cigarettes were first marketed in the United States in 2007. The use of these products in adolescence was recently reviewed in the journal of the American Medical association, *JAMA Pediatrics*, involving a very large sample size. The researchers concluded:

Use of e-cigarettes was associated with higher odds of ever or current cigarette smoking, higher odds of established smoking, higher odds of planning to quit smoking among current smokers, and, among experimenters, lower odds of abstinence from conventional cigarettes. Use of e- cigarettes does not discourage, and may encourage, conventional cigarette use among U.S. adolescents. (Dutra and Glantz 2014, Conclusions and Relevance)

There are also reports that this vehicle is being used as a delivery system for other drugs. For example, marijuana used in liquid and wax forms does not generate the typical marijuana odour.

Alcoholics are more likely to die from tobacco-related causes than from the direct effect of alcohol. The rate of smoking among alcoholics is three times higher than the general public, and that's true whether the alcoholic is still practising or in recovery. Between 80 and 95 percent of alcoholics smoke cigarettes and approximately 70 percent of alcoholics are heavy smokers (more than one package per day). The rate of tobacco smoking among drug addicts is estimated to be about the same (Richter et al., 2002).

In spite of these figures, treatment programs have been reluctant to include nicotine abstinence as a goal of treatment. Typical concerns include the impression that this would overload patients already giving up alcohol and other drugs — it would be too much for them. And perhaps patients would not enter treatment if smoking cessation were required. Research has not been extensive in this area, but a review of the issue in an article entitled "Smoking Cessation and Alcohol Abstinence: What Do the Data Tell Us?" (Gulliver et al. 2006) suggests that abstaining from smoking/nicotine leads to more positive outcomes in terms of long-term sobriety, and conversely, that continued smoking increases the risk of relapse for alcoholics.

Alcohol

With the exception of nicotine, alcohol is widely available and remains the most common addiction. It has a variety of neurotransmitter targets, however it primarily exerts its action in the brain through something called GABA receptors. Known as "inhibitory neurotransmitters," these mechanisms act to calm the system down. They also happen to be where benzodiazepines exert their action, although in a somewhat different spot on the GABA receptor. GABA receptors have an important relationship with another neurotransmitter, glutamate, which generally has the opposite effect. It is stimulatory. Under normal conditions, these two neurotransmitters are in balance with each other. Think of a teeter-totter in a neutral position. When alcoholics drink on a regular basis, the GABA system is more activated (it becomes the heavyweight on the teeter-totter) relative to the glutamate system, keeping things more calmed down and sedated. In a detoxification setting, when alcoholics are withdrawing, the balance swings in the opposite direction and glutamate becomes overactive system (it is now the heavyweight on the teeter-totter), leading to typical withdrawal symptoms.

Sedatives (Benzodiazepines, Barbiturates, "Z Drugs")

Benzodiazepines are a group of medications generally used for anxiety and insomnia treatment. Best-known examples include diazepam, known as Valium; lorazepam, known as Ativan; clonazepam, known as Rivotril; and alprazolam, known as Xanax. All are generally indicated for short-term use only. A very important difference between benzodiazepines is their duration of action. Some are more short-acting, with an action that only lasts a few hours; long-acting benzodiazepines last much longer. In general, short-acting benzodiazepines tend to be more addictive and are harder to detoxify from. While still addictive, long-acting benzodiazepines are less so, and have a smoother withdrawal. For this reason, patients addicted to very high-dose, short-acting benzodiazepines are typically switched to long-acting ones for the purpose of withdrawal.

Many people can take these medications for long-term management of anxiety without becoming addicted. But if one has a risk for addiction generally, one can become addicted to these medications, and they can be extremely difficult to get off of. In the past, barbiturates were prescribed to manage anxiety and insomnia but they are rarely used these days. However, Fiorinal, a pain medication that has been used for migraine headaches, does contain a barbiturate, which can lead to seizures on withdrawal if not managed properly.

Benzodiazepines and barbiturates have withdrawal symptoms very similar to alcohol—including seizures and, possibly, death—and need to be managed appropriately (see chapter 7, Detoxification).

Imovane (zopiclone) and Ambien (zolpidem) were initially marketed as nonaddictive medications. They are still often thought of as such. However, their use has escalated over the last several years, and it has become clear that that addiction does occur with these "Z drugs," as they are sometimes called.

GHB deserves some special discussion. It is an illicit drug typically used in a binge fashion, and is often associated with after-hour parties. However, on occasion, one comes across a daily heavy user of GHB. It has withdrawal effects very similar to alcohol and is treated in a similar fashion. Serious withdrawal problems including seizures have been observed.

Opiates

Opiates are a family of drugs primarily used for pain management. There are numerous semisynthetic (e.g., hydromorphone, oxycodone, hydrocodone) and synthetic opiates (e.g., fentanyl, methadone, tramadol) in this class. Naturally occurring forms, including morphine, codeine, and the street drug heroin, are derived from the opium plant. In the past, heroin was the most prevalent opiate of abuse. It has now been replaced by a variety of prescription opiates, although heroin remains widely available and is generally cheaper than prescription opiates. In a common scenario, some individuals abuse or are dependent on prescription opiates. When they lack access to their prescription opiate of choice, or money to purchase a prescription, they then turn to heroin and subsequently become addicted to it.

Opiates exert their action through opiate receptors in the brain and elsewhere in the body. Opiate receptors can be activated either by external agents such as opiate medications, or other internal substances that act on the same receptors. A well-known example is the runner's high. When runners run, their bodies produce an opiate called endorphin, which acts on the opiate receptors and generates a high of sorts.

Use of opiates causes a variety of effects including the classic pinpoint pupils and constipation. Methadone and buprenorphine, both long-acting opiates, are used to stabilize heroin addiction and prescription opiate addictions.

Prescription opiates, both short-acting and long-acting, are primarily available in the community as tablets. These tablets are obviously meant for swallowing and absorption through the gut. Addicts have discovered, however, that the tablets can be crushed and snorted for a much more rapid and robust effect. They can also be dissolved and injected. Many long-acting tablets have their long duration of effect as a result of the coating on the tablet. When the pill is crushed and snorted it becomes a short-acting opiate and therefore withdrawal typically comes on more quickly.

There has been a dramatic escalation in the last few years of deaths from accidental overdoses from prescription opiates and heroin (see chapter 8, Hot Topics, for more on this). Death comes from the respiratory system shutting down. This happens when people take excessive amounts of opiates, relative to their tolerance. As discussed above, tolerance develops when people continue to use drugs — in this case, prescription opiates: that is, they require more and more of the drug to get the same effect.

The whole issue of tolerance is extremely important. Opiate users will lose their tolerance when they stop using or cut back significantly. If they return to use at the same level at which they stopped, they no longer have the same tolerance and can die from accidental overdose. In addition, street drugs can be sold with a range of purity and can also be misrepresented. When one buys drugs from street sources, quality control is lost. In a common recent example in British Columbia, drugs described as OxyContin are sold, yet they actually contain fentanyl, which is many times more potent than heroin; this in itself can lead to accidental overdose.

Stimulants (Cocaine, Crack Cocaine, Methamphetamine)

Stimulants such as cocaine, crack cocaine, and methamphetamine act on the brain to dramatically increase dopamine levels well above the normal ranges experienced in daily life. This is experienced as a profound euphoria. Prescription stimulants such as Dexedrine and Ritalin also raise dopamine levels, but at a much slower rate and to a much lesser extent. (Their action can be boosted by crushing and snorting.)

Cocaine and methamphetamine are often sold in small packets or gram quantities. A slang term used in cocaine addiction is an "eight ball" — a 3.5 gram packet, or "eighth of an ounce." Alcohol and cocaine are often used together. People often drink to the point of intoxication and use cocaine to counter these effects—to sober up. When alcohol and cocaine are used together, a unique metabolite (cocaethylene) is formed, which generally has a longer action than cocaine alone. As cocaine use progresses, the switch is often made from powder cocaine to crack cocaine, and then on occasion to intravenous use.

Ecstasy, MDMA

Ecstasy is the name originally given to MDMA. In reality, Ecstasy is frequently a heavily adulterated formulation by the time it hits the streets. Samples of Ecstasy which have been taken from after-hour parties and raves often find a large mix of adulterants, and users often differentiate these drugs as a result. The drug is used primarily in after-hour parties, often together with various other drugs. It tends to have some stimulant properties as well as significant hallucinogenic/psychedelic effects. Users may experience clenching of the jaw and grinding of the teeth as well as dry mouth. Onset of action is typically a half hour to an hour, peaking within one and a half hours to two hours for total high of three or four hours.

Marijuana

Marijuana and hashish, which contain the resin from the marijuana plant, act on cannabinoid receptors in the brain where they exert their action, generating their high. Cannabinoid receptors are also widely distributed throughout the body, and therefore have a number of other actions beyond euphoria. The high is caused primarily by the THC, the most active ingredient in marijuana. THC concentration has increased over the last several years through genetic enhancement. (See a detailed discussion of issues surrounding medical marijuana in chapter 13, Hot Topics.)

Synthetic Cannabis

Synthetic cannabinoids are psychoactive designer drugs, which may go by the brand name K2 or Spice. One of the challenges of law enforcement is that street chemists continually modify known psychoactive drugs that are currently illegal to generate new drugs that are not covered by current laws. As a result, synthetic cannabinoid drugs can be created which slip through the net and can be legally marketed. These drugs are often marketed as if for other purposes — such as incense or air freshener — but end up being used as a form of marijuana. Interestingly, synthetic cannabis does not produce positive results in drug tests for THC, although it can be specifically tested for. Attempts have been made to expedite the laws to enhance enforcement, although apparently this has been very difficult. Synthetic cannabinoids appear to be more toxic and have more significant adverse effects, including death (Synthetic Cannabinoids 2013).

Hallucinogens

Experimentation in adolescence with LSD and magic mushrooms is common in the history of people who later develop serious addictions. Recently, the use of salvia has become increasingly common.

Salvia is an herb in the sage family. It is typically smoked and has a very short duration of action. It has a hallucinogenic/psychedelic effect and is most commonly used in the late teenage years. It is reportedly easily accessible in Canada and has been the subject of various media reports, including a recent documentary on CTV W5 (Derrick 2013).

Ketamine

In the past, ketamine was used as an anesthetic agent, particularly in veterinary medicine, and was generally available on a very limited basis, through diversion from legitimate supplies. More recently, clandestine laboratories have been making ketamine illegally, increasing access to the drug in North America. Some individuals use ketamine to enhance a spiritual experience, as the drug characteristically causes a feeling of detachment from one's physical body and the external world. DXM (dextromethorphan), a cough suppressant component in some cough syrups, has similar effects when taken in large doses.

Ketamine has become a significant focus of research in the area of psychiatry. Several proof-of-concept studies have been made using intravenous, intramuscular, and nasal spray formulations of low-dose ketamine for the treatment of very severe and refractory depression as well as posttraumatic stress disorder (Feder et al. 2014). These studies have demonstrated rapid and robust improvements, although the benefits may be time-limited. The studies are of particular interest in psychiatry, as ketamine acts on different neurotransmitter systems than typical antidepressants, opening up potential therapeutic targets in the future. There are several recent reviews in the medical literature (Chang et al. 2013).

Chapter 4

Diagnosing Addiction

Diagnosis: The Three Cs

Specialists often speak of the three Cs of addiction: *compulsion, control,* and *consequences. Compulsion* refers to the very powerful drive to obtain and use substances. This drive includes obsessive thoughts as well as compulsive behaviours. I recall a professional woman, in her thirties, who was in treatment for her addiction to crack cocaine. She described an increasing preoccupation with using crack cocaine as her work day progressed. By the end of the afternoon her thoughts were almost entirely consumed by her desire to use crack cocaine. She would take the bus home with increasing impatience. Finally, she would literally sprint to her front door and almost immediately begin using and experienced a major reduction in tension.

Addicts experience a loss of *control* over their use of the substance or behaviour in question. One of the hallmarks of addiction is that people repeatedly and progressively break their own rules about how or when they will use their substance. Commonly, they may promise themselves not to drink until a certain time of day, not to drink and drive, not to drink every day, not to drink while their children require attention and supervision, and not to use alcohol or drugs in the workplace or in ways that interfere with their work function.

Many negative *consequences* attend the continued behaviour or use of the substance. Addicts commonly lose significant relationships and experience such things as medical complications, legal difficulties, health concerns, and work-related impairments.

The *Diagnostic and Statistical Manual of Mental Disorders* (DSM-5), now in its fifth edition, is the most widely accepted reference used by clinicians and researchers for classifying mental disorders in North America. It provides several criteria for making a diagnosis of substance use disorder that incorporate the three Cs (see table 2).

The fourth edition of the DSM broke down addiction into *abuse* and *dependence*. In contrast, the DSM-5 speaks of substance use disorders of mild, moderate, or severe intensity. It was felt that the term *dependence* was confusing, as one could be physiologically dependent on different substances and yet not be addicted. Classic examples included dependence on prescription opiates, benzodiazepines, and even a number of antidepressants. Many individuals use these medications in a stable manner, as prescribed, and show none of the obvious symptoms of addiction. However, when use of the medication is abruptly discontinued, withdrawal symptoms do emerge.

Behavioural Addictions

Patients who are treated for substance use disorders will often displace their addiction from chemicals onto other addictive behaviours that manifest the three Cs. They may also exclusively manifest a behavioural addiction in the absence of a substance use disorder. The term *behavioural addiction* has been used to describe some of these behaviours. Common examples include sexually addictive behaviour; addictive spending, shopping, videogame playing, and gambling; and various forms of Internet addiction. These

Table 2
DSM-5 Criteria for Diagnosing Substance Use Disorders

1.	Taking the substance in larger amounts or for longer than originally intended
2.	Expressing a persistent desire to cut down or regulate substance use, but reporting multiple unsuccessful efforts to decrease or discontinue use
3.	Spending a great deal of time obtaining the substance, using the substance, or recovering from its effects
4.	Craving, manifested by an intense desire or urge for the drug; may occur at any time but more likely when in an environment where the drug previously was obtained or used
5.	Failing to fulfill major role obligations at work, school, or home, due to recurrent substance use
6.	Continuing to use, despite having persistent or recurrent social or interpersonal problems caused or exacerbated by the effects of the substance
7.	Giving up or reducing important social, occupational, or recreational activities because of substance use; may include withdrawing from family activities and hobbies
8.	Using over and over again, even in situations in which it is physically hazardous
9.	Continuing to use, despite knowing that a persistent or recurrent physical or psychological problem is likely to have been caused or exacerbated by the substance
10.	Requiring a markedly increased dose of the substance to achieve the desired effect or a markedly reduced effect when the usual dose is consumed; tolerance
11.	Developing withdrawal symptoms that can be relieved by taking more of the substance

Scoring:
- No diagnosis: 0 or 1 criterion met
- Mild substance use disorder: 2 to 3 criteria met
- Moderate substance use disorder: 4 to 5 criteria met
- Severe substance use disorder: 6 or more criteria met

disorders are all characterized by a compulsion to engage in the behaviour, associated with loss of control and negative consequences. Like substance use disorders, behavioural addictions are often triggered by various emotional states or life events. Most addiction treatment programs consider them to be addiction disorders and clinically treat them as such. Twelve-step programs are generally available for most of these behavioural addictions.

The DSM-5 names gambling disorder as a behavioural addiction. Serious consideration was given to including hypersexual disorder (what addiction workers would generally describe as sex addiction), but it was felt that there was not adequate evidence to include it at this time. Internet gaming disorder was placed in an appendix, indicating that further study was required. The DSM-5 has subsumed various eating disorders under the category of Feeding and Eating Disorders, including anorexia nervosa, bulimia nervosa, and most recently, binge-eating disorder in the list (see chapter 9, Concurrent Disorders, for a further discussion of this topic).

Sexuality and Addiction

When the DSM-5 was being revised, consideration was given to including what many in the addiction field would describe as sexual addiction. Criteria were proposed for *hypersexual disorder*. This proposed disorder was eventually excluded from the DSM-5 on the basis that there was not enough research available to include it. Nevertheless, I am including the proposed criteria for hypersexual disorder here.

Proposed criteria for hypersexual disorder. Over a period of at least six months, a person experiences clinically significant personal distress or impairment in social, occupational, or other important areas of functioning, associated with the frequency and intensity of the sexual fantasies, urges, and behaviour. These sexual fantasies, urges, and behaviour may include masturbation, cybersex, pornography viewing, telephone sex, strip clubs, and sexual behaviour with consenting adults, among others. They are not due to direct physiological effects of drugs or medications, or to manic episodes. The person experiences recurrent and intense sexual fantasies, sexual urges, and sexual behaviour in association with four or more of the following five criteria:

1. Consuming excessive time with sexual fantasies and urges, and planning for and engaging in sexual behaviour.

2. Repetitively engaging in sexual fantasies, urges, and behaviour in response to dysphoric mood states, such as anxiety, depression, boredom, and irritability.

3. Repetitively engaging in sexual fantasies, urges, and behaviour in response to stressful life events.

4. Repetitively but unsuccessfully attempting to control or significantly reduce the sexual fantasies, urges, and behaviour.

5. Repetitively engaging in sexual behaviour while disregarding the risk for physical or emotional harm to self or others.

The three Cs (compulsion, control, and consequences) are clearly evident in the criteria for this addiction disorder. The compulsive nature of the behaviours with associated loss of control and negative consequences are also evident.

Relationship between addiction and sexuality. Childhood sexual abuse is frequently observed in the developmental history of many men and women who struggle with a substance use disorder. This is obviously a significant trauma and may initiate a pattern of subsequently acting out in sexual areas, which may express itself in the form of promiscuity, sexual identity issues, or sexual avoidance. People with substance use disorders also commonly report having been sexually assaulted in the past. These assaults have often occurred in the context of intoxication and blackouts, and as a result, people may or may not recollect the traumatic events. Many survivors of sexual assault blame themselves because of their intoxication, and need reassurance to understand that being intoxicated was not an invitation to sexual violence.

Sexual behaviours may be a mechanism to generate money to support a drug habit. This may include escorting, prostitution, exotic dancing, or exchanging sex for drugs. For male addicts in new communities, finding escorts or prostitutes can be a reliable way of accessing drugs.

Users of cocaine, crack cocaine, and methamphetamine frequently use these stimulant drugs in association with various sexual behaviours. They may use while engaged in sexual behaviours with their own partners, or they may purchase drugs to use with escorts or prostitutes. Many addicts have described using cocaine or crack and spending hours masturbating to pornography on the Internet or videos. As the addiction progresses and the use of drugs escalates, it is not uncommon for the interest in sex to drop off. Where stimulants in early use may enhance sexual performance, addicts often complain of loss of performance as their addiction progresses. As noted in Jake's case, described in chapter 8, gay men are frequently known to make contact and amplify the experience through the use of methamphetamine. There appears to be a somewhat increased prevalence of methamphetamine use in the gay, lesbian, and transgendered communities.

Sexually addictive behaviours can be a primary and exclusive issue, or comorbid with various other substance use disorders. They can involve sexual relationships with multiple partners; compulsive use of pornography online; or other forms or engaging in repetitive, high-risk behaviours. Patrick Carnes (2001, 2002) has written extensively in the area of sexually addictive behaviours, including online addiction. (Also, see the case study of Jake, in chapter 10.)

There are various twelve-step treatment approaches to sexually addictive behaviours. One of the challenging problems relates to the issue of abstinence. Long-term abstinence is not a realistic goal, as one might expect with alcohol and drugs. Instead the goal may be changed to managing sexual behaviours within a healthy range.

CASE STUDY: MICHAEL

Michael's case clearly demonstrates the three C's of addiction, as well as severe cocaine/crack cocaine use disorder and alcohol use disorder, and some elements of behavioural addiction.[1]

Michael, forty-nine, was employed by a well-known telecommunications company. He was employed in a position where safety issues were critical for himself, coworkers, and the public. He had been single for several years, but before that had been married twice. He had a sixteen-year-old son with whom he had had minimal contact in the last decade. He was isolated and

---

[1] In all the case studies in this book, various clinical details have been omitted or altered in order to protect the confidentiality of our patients.

had few social contacts. His job and livelihood were at risk and his relapse potential was significant.

Michael's treatment for alcohol and cocaine/crack cocaine dependence was mandated by his employer, following an intervention after his serious addiction to these substances came to the employer's attention. He stopped using for almost six weeks following the intervention, but suffered a relapse after which he came into treatment. He admitted to alcohol problems going back to his teenage years. From the age of thirteen until he was twenty-two, he had been a heavy binge drinker. He lost his driver's licence, would get into fights, and eventually ended up in prison briefly. At twenty-two, he began using cocaine and for many years used cocaine after he finished work, staying up until the wee hours of the morning. He would be exhausted for work the next day, although he felt he was effective at hiding his addiction from others. By the age of twenty-seven he was using cocaine regularly and by the time he was thirty-five to forty-two, he started using large amounts of cocaine during the day while at work, switching to drinking in the evenings at least a few times a week. At the age of forty-two he switched to freebasing cocaine (converting powdered cocaine to a smokable form), as his nasal mucosa were deteriorating from snorting the drug. He also described significant sexually addictive behaviours, associated with his use of cocaine and crack. He still drank heavily now, at least a few days a week; he never went more than three days without alcohol. He had not had any significant periods of abstinence with the exception of going into detox in 2005 for approximately two weeks, followed by forty days of residential treatment. He had relapsed three hours after leaving treatment at that time. His difficulties had continued to progress, becoming increasingly problematic in the previous year.

Michael had no significant psychiatric history other than mood swings secondary to his addiction. He described a very strong family history of addiction, including two maternal uncles, a paternal grandfather, and a brother who were alcoholic. He was not aware of any mental illness or suicides in the family.

He did not require detoxification at the time of admission. Based on medical assessments on admission, he was diagnosed with alcohol, cocaine, and nicotine use disorders/severe under the DSM-5.

In treatment, Michael appeared to recognize the seriousness of his situation and was motivated to address his addiction. He worked through his assignments without difficulty. He recognized that addiction had controlled his life for many years. He discussed his shame and guilt related to his progressive addiction. He tended to be distracted by outside concerns, particularly his relationship with his family and employer. This made it difficult for him to focus "one day at a time" on getting well. Phone conferences with his employer provided additional support and allowed him to let this go. On the basis of the severity and longevity of his addiction, he was transferred to the extended-care program for continuing treatment. During the course of treatment, he was increasingly able to identify his feelings and emotions and communicate these with others. He was also able to take and give honest feedback to assist himself and others with recovery.

Michael completed treatment and was discharged with a number of aftercare recommendations in addition to the employer's protocol for drug testing and aftercare requirements. Michael was in treatment for a total of five months. Based on available information, it would appear that he stayed clean and sober for approximately six months. However, he began to reduce his commitment to the recovery process and relapsed to alcohol. His employer was aware of this and said they would follow an appropriate course of action. This might involve being readmitted for treatment, terminating his employment, or tightening up his outpatient process follow-up by having him go to more twelve-step meetings, attend more appointments with this counsellor or physician, and undergo more random drug screens.

Chapter 5

Screening for Addiction

We all go to the family doctor for various medical and health issues. People may also go to counsellors, health practitioners, clergy, and psychiatrists. These helpers need to be able to identify alcohol or drug addiction in its early stages, before it gets to the point that people face serious consequences or require residential treatment.

According to National Institute on Alcohol Abuse and Alcoholism research, only 14.6 percent of people with alcohol abuse or dependence receive treatment (NIAAA 2010). While a significant number of these people will improve without treatment (White 2012), a hope or belief that they can "do it by themselves" — a form of denial — may only serve to keep them from getting help. Shame, guilt, and the associated stigma of seeking assistance for alcohol dependence or addiction will also keep people in their alcohol or drug-related isolation.

Health care professionals are in a unique position to identify addiction disorders in their clients and patients. Patients often present with numerous problems, while hiding an underlying addiction disorder. Common examples include insomnia, anxiety, depression, gastrointestinal complaints, sexual dysfunction, marital tension and family issues, falls and injuries, and work-related absences. If screening and assessment for addiction is not a part of clinicians' routine practice, they will inevitably fail to identify patients with addiction and miss the opportunity to assist.

Screening for addiction disorders can range from a simple discussion about alcohol and drug use to a much more structured or standardized assessment approach. It is critical to recall that alcoholics come in all shapes and sizes, and from every socioeconomic level; and the majority continue to function in their work settings until the disease is very advanced. Don't let your stereotype of an alcoholic cause you to miss appropriately screening and treating a patient or client!

A few of these approaches are discussed below. All are available online.

The CAGE Questionnaire

CAGE is a questionnaire commonly used in screening for addiction ("CAGE questionnaire" n.d.). C is for *cutting down*: clients or patients are asked whether they have made any attempts to cut down or control their use of alcohol or drugs in the past. A is for the defensive *anger* that addicts respond with, when questioned about their alcohol consumption. G is for the *guilt* related to things that addicts have done or not done as a result of their drinking. E is for the *eyeopener:* the drink that alcoholics take first thing in the morning to relieve withdrawal symptoms so they will "feel normal" and be able to function during the day.

A positive response to the CAGE questionnaire, particularly when two or more positives are found, suggests a significant risk for alcohol use disorder. Collateral information from a family member or friend may also be very helpful in diagnosing substance use disorders. Asking if a partner, spouse, or friend has been concerned about their drinking may also raise important flags.

Structured Screening Instruments

A number of useful, validated questionnaires can assist in identifying patients with substance use disorders (SAMHSA n.d.). The Michigan alcohol screening test (MAST) is a practical screening questionnaire which can be used in an office setting for diagnosis of alcohol dependence. The alcohol use disorders identification test (AUDIT) is another commonly used example. The drug abuse screening test (DAST), is available for diagnosing drug addictions. Similar questionnaires are available, such as the CRAFFT, designed specifically for youth, and others designed to ask about marijuana use. These screening tests are all available online.

Helping Patients Who Drink Too Much:
A Clinician's Guide

The NIAAA has developed an important tool, *Helping Patients Who Drink Too Much: A Clinician's Guide* (NIAAA n.d.). The online resource also includes videotaped demonstrations applying this process to patients in different settings and with different levels of severity of alcohol dependence. The program is a four-step model:

- Step 1: Ask about alcohol use
- Step 2: Assess for alcohol use disorders
- Step 3: Advise and assist
- Step 4: Follow-up and continue support

Step 1 starts with the simple question, "Do you sometimes drink beer, wine or other alcoholic beverages?" Screening is complete if the answer is No. If the answer is Yes, the following question is then asked: "How many times in the past year have you had five or more drinks in a day (for men), or four or more drinks in a day (for women)?"

If these thresholds have not been exceeded, the patient or client is advised to stay within maximum drinking limits for healthy men—no more than four drinks in a day AND no more than fourteen drinks in a week; for healthy women, no more than three drinks in a day AND no more than seven drinks in a week. These levels have generally been correlated with safe drinking. When alcohol is consumed regularly in levels above the recommended guidelines, research suggests a risk of negative medical consequences increases.

Similar guidelines are available in many countries, although the maximum drinking limits vary somewhat from country to country. British Columbia, Canada has instituted a similar guideline ("Problem drinking" 2013).

If the screening was positive for one or more heavy drinking days in the past year, further questions about the amount of alcohol consumed are asked, focusing on numbers of days of the week when alcohol is taken and in what typical quantities. The screening then proceeds to Step 2.

Step 2 reviews the DSM-5 criteria to determine whether a possible diagnosis of alcohol use disorder can be made. If so, treatment recommendations are reviewed and discussed. If an alcohol use disorder is not present, the concept of risk and safe drinking are then reviewed. Determination is made as to the patient's or client's willingness to commit to changes and a specific plan is discussed. These will be followed up later (Steps 3 and 4; chapters 7–10 of this book cover treatment in depth.)

These brief alcohol interventions in primary health care settings, as they have been called, have been well documented to be effective for addressing hazardous and harmful drinking, particularly in middle-aged male drinkers. This is confirmed in a recent systematic review (O'Donnell et al. 2014).

Laboratory Investigation

Patients with substance use disorders frequently minimize or lie about the extent of their drinking or drug use. This is important for clinicians to keep in mind when assessing someone initially as well as when assessing for relapse after periods of sobriety. Laboratory investigation is therefore another useful tool for assessing and diagnosing substance use disorders.

Laboratory test results may reflect heavier use than patients or clients are reporting. For example, alcohol is toxic to certain blood cells. A complete blood count may reveal enlarged red blood cells and a reduced number of platelets if they have been drinking heavily. As is well known, alcohol is also toxic to the liver. Damage to the liver can be evaluated by using common liver function tests for such indicators as GGT, AST, ALT, and bilirubin (Lazo and Clark 2011).

A urine sample may identify specific drugs that the patient has not reported taking, or indicate relapse following a period of sobriety. Another use of drug testing is to confirm that a patient is actually taking any addictive medication that has been prescribed. This may identify patients who are selling their prescribed medication to others rather than taking it themselves.

Chapter 6

Getting into Treatment

Substance use disorders tend to be progressive, with the fallout expanding in ever-larger circles. The rate of progress can be very gradual, even over decades, although sometimes it can happen with frightening speed. Ultimately, even with the best of attempts to keep things hidden, the fact that there is a serious problem becomes increasingly evident. Still, one of the most challenging issues in the field of addiction is how to persuade someone with an addiction to go for help as early in the process as possible. Family members often feel that they can only stand by, powerless to intervene, watching as loved ones continue to deteriorate. How can this progressive deterioration be addressed? In our experience, there are several ways.

Initiated by Oneself

In the end, all attempts to quit drinking or using drugs must be centred and grounded in oneself. Some people choose to do it solo; others choose to reach out and ask for help. Whether on their own or with others, however, in the best-case scenario they recognize that they have a problem and make a choice to halt the addictive behaviour. They get to the point that they are "sick and tired of being sick and tired" and make the decision to quit drinking or using drugs so they can feel better.

Pregnancy can be an ideal time to address addiction—I have seen several women discover that they are pregnant and choose to stop using drugs during the course of their pregnancy. Sometimes, people just recognize that their physical health is deteriorating, or they become worried about their finances, or they realize that significant relationships are threatened; then they quit on their own. The next obvious challenge is to "stay quit."

Motivated by Friends

Close friends may well bear witness to the significant changes in a person's emotional state or behaviour as their addiction progresses. In my experience, the willingness of a close friend(s) to sit down and have an honest discussion about their concerns can be a significant factor in the decision to seek help. It is not uncommon for this initial expression of concern to be met with a response of defensiveness and anger, but it can also be lifesaving—it is equally possible that the response will be one of relief: "the cat's out of the bag," freeing the person to be honest about their problems.

The Family As Part of the Problem and Part of the Solution

All too often, family members are left watching helplessly as their loved ones are devoured by addiction. Everything changes—their loved ones' physical health deteriorates, they become increasingly isolated, and their moodiness and anger only increases. Parents watch their children become homeless, without food or shelter, living on the streets or couch surfing in various friends' homes. Family relationships become strained, and everyone is affected. Often, loved ones may steal and pawn family items and even resort to the significant manipulation of threatening suicide. So the family does everything in its power to rescue them. But any such rescue attempts are foiled. The loved ones continue their demands for money, or for the opportunity to live at home again—when they have already been asked to leave so many times, because of the total disruption and chaos they created when they lived at home in the past.

There is considerable literature related to the family consequences of addiction and the development of codependency. Because addiction often runs in families, these same family members may have grown up in alcoholic families and have taken on a caregiver role from a very early age. They have been trained to put others' needs ahead of their own and often became their parent's parent.

Assisting the family to establish healthy boundaries, and coaching them to respond to the addict, can be a very helpful intervention. Even if a patient is initially not willing to get help, appropriate interventions with family members can lead to a more positive outcome.

Helped by Health Care Professionals

As noted in chapter 5, patients often present to health professionals with a variety of concerns. When health professionals understand addiction and use appropriate screening, they can help identify addiction disorders and then find appropriate intervention approaches.

Jump-Started by Interventionists

In the field of addictions, there are professionals whose job is to work with family members and friends to perform interventions with people suffering from an addiction disorder. This has been popularized in the A&E television reality show, *Intervention*, and more recently in the Canadian series, *Intervention Canada*. Different styles of interventions are used. Commonly, an interventionist will meet ahead of time with family members, friends, and other significant key players to gather information on the identified person, and participants are asked to write letters that they will read at the intervention. They are instructed that their initial tone is to be loving and supportive, while clearly stating their concerns and observations regarding addiction. After the letters are read, the identified person is invited to go immediately to a prearranged treatment centre. All is prepared in advance, including travel arrangements.

If the identified person refuses to accept the offer, the next phase of the intervention might be for the attendees to read a letter outlining the consequences. These may involve suspending the relationship, refusing to offer further financial or housing assistance, or setting other boundaries to prevent being further negatively impacted by the identified person's addiction. That person's emotional responses to the intervention vary widely, from anger and walking out to a powerful sense of relief and gratitude. Generally, response rates are very positive and the intervention is profoundly impacting.

Mandated by Employers

Many employers, particularly in larger corporations, have developed alcohol and drug policies to identify and assist employees with substance use disorders. Such employees are typically referred to a specialist for independent assessment, and recommendations follow. Many companies have an employee assistance program, that offers counselling and referral. Residential treatment is often requested for employees with more severe addiction disorders, particularly if they are working in safety-sensitive positions.

Chapter 7

Withdrawal, Assessment, and Tools for Treatment

One of the most important things to consider when deciding to quit drinking or using drugs is the medical risk associated with withdrawal. A medical professional should always be consulted. Suddenly stopping daily use of alcohol, benzodiazepines, barbiturates, or GHB can lead to seizures and even death. On the other hand, stopping opiate use is generally not considered dangerous. However, it is extremely uncomfortable and is best managed under medical supervision.

In this chapter I review the process of withdrawing from addictive substances and offer information on treatment options beyond withdrawal. People can withdraw in community settings, but here I concentrate on the process of withdrawal in the more intensive settings, including detoxification units, treatment centres, and hospitals.

Withdrawal

As their addictive disease spirals out of control, people may feel trapped. They know they can no longer continue using but, equally, they fear stopping because of the risks and discomfort associated with withdrawal. This is particularly true for alcohol and prescription opiate users, but also applies to people who use benzodiazepines and possibly GHB. They arrive for treatment in various states, ranging from abstinence to acute intoxication to severe withdrawal. Accurate assessment of the withdrawal requirements are critical in establishing safety and a trusting relationship with the patient. Safely withdrawing patients begins with this initial contact.

Establishing where patients will be treated is one of the first concerns. Low-risk patients with mild withdrawal symptoms can be managed on an outpatient basis. Conversely, patients with complex medical problems, or at high risk of medical complications during the withdrawal process, may require a hospital setting in order to ensure a safe withdrawal process. The American Society of Addiction Medicine (ASAM) has addressed this issue in its placement and treatment criteria (Mee-Lee 2001, 2013). For purposes of determining appropriate treatment settings, they have identified several important factors, known as the six dimensions of multidimensional assessment:

1. Acute intoxication/withdrawal
2. Biomedical factors
3. Psychiatric factors
4. Treatment acceptance/resistance
5. Relapse/continued use potential
6. Recovery/living environment

Each of the six dimensions is associated with an estimated range of severity, on a scale from 1 to 4.

Taking these six factors into account, ASAM has identified five levels of care for withdrawal management:

Level 1:   Ambulatory withdrawal management without extended on-site monitoring
Level 2:   As above, with extended on-site monitoring

Level 3:   Social detoxification — clinically managed residential withdrawal management
Level 4:   Medical detoxification unit — medically monitored inpatient withdrawal management
Level 5:   Medically managed intensive inpatient withdrawal management

The six factors are very important variables in deciding what settings are most appropriate. For example, an alcoholic who is a heavy daily drinker with a history of alcohol withdrawal seizures and known heart disease, who is currently very depressed and suicidal, and who has limited family support, will need a much more intensive medically supervised setting for withdrawal than a heavy crack cocaine user, because safety issues related to cocaine withdrawal are minimal.

At Edgewood, patients who are withdrawing from various substances are immediately integrated with other patients in treatment. There is no separate area or program for patients who are withdrawing. Modifications may be made depending on individualized need, but generally patients are expected to follow the daytime structure of activities as much as possible. Some patients clearly find this difficult and would prefer to be in bed or isolated from other patients. At Edgewood, we believe that it is important to counter this preference; our stance is that patients in withdrawal should begin to make connections right away with other patients, who are able to provide support. Particularly if they have been in withdrawal themselves in the recent past, they can be a source of optimism and encouragement.

Other settings (such as withdrawal management units) may have minimal daytime structure during the acute withdrawal phase. It is important to note that withdrawal alone is NOT treatment for addiction and should always be followed with treatment of the addiction disorder.

Alcohol

Alcohol generally remains the most common drug that people need medical help to withdraw from. It is extremely important to evaluate the clinical state of all new patients and determine their risk for withdrawal-related complications.

Withdrawal

Generally speaking, the risk of significant alcohol withdrawal increases with duration of drinking; quantity of alcohol consumed; prior history of alcohol withdrawal problems in the past; or a history of significant alcohol withdrawal symptoms in the morning, requiring a morning eyeopener.

As people continue to drink alcohol on a daily basis, they develop tolerance and dependence. If they suddenly stop drinking, they may experience acute withdrawal symptoms: tremors, nausea and vomiting, sweating, anxiety, insomnia, increased blood pressure, and increased heart rate. This typically begins within six to twelve hours of quitting drinking. As withdrawal progresses there is a risk of seizures, typically within twenty-four to forty-eight hours after stopping drinking. Untreated in chronic alcohol users, this trend may progress toward the risk of a syndrome called delirium tremens (DTs). (This term is often applied incorrectly. Early symptoms of alcohol withdrawal are not DTs.) The "delirium" in delirium tremens means being extremely disoriented as to person, place, and time. People in DTs may experience profound confusion, and may also experience visual and auditory hallucinations. This syndrome typically occurs following three to five days of abstinence from alcohol.

Untreated, such patients may die as a result of hyperthermia, cardiac stress, or dehydration.

Treatment

Evaluation is typically assisted by the use of various standardized assessment tools. The most commonly used tool for measuring the severity of alcohol withdrawal is CIWA, the Clinical Institute Withdrawal Assessment — Alcohol (Centre for Addiction and Mental Health 2001). This scale is commonly used in hospital and medical withdrawal settings.

Three widely used approaches for treatment of alcohol withdrawal are symptom-triggered therapy, fixed-schedule therapy, and front-end loading.

Symptom-triggered therapy. This approach is individualized in response to need. Benzodiazepines, typically either diazepam (Valium) or lorazepam (Ativan), are administered in direct proportion to the CIWA score, at intervals varying with the severity of the withdrawal risk. Thiamine (vitamin B1) is also administered. The advantage of this approach is that only the amount of medication that is necessary is given, based on objective measurement. Staff who are trained in this approach are required, along with well-established protocols and close monitoring.

Fixed-schedule therapy. In fixed-schedule therapy, patients are determined to be low-, moderate-, or high-dose candidates, based on risk assessment at the time of admission. They are placed on a light, standard, or heavy detoxification protocol using a benzodiazepine, usually Valium or Ativan. CIWA scales are assessed at least four times daily in order to measure the response to treatment. Medications are gradually tapered off over a period of approximately one week. Thiamine is always administered as well. This is generally a very practical and manageable approach.

A recent study compared the fixed-schedule approach with the symptom-triggered approach for uncomplicated alcohol withdrawal. It found that the amounts of medications administered and the duration of treatment were both significantly less with symptom-triggered therapy (Sachdeva et al. 2014).

Front-end loading. This third, less common, approach is a much more aggressive treatment. It is particularly effective for rapidly stabilizing withdrawal symptoms in high-risk patients. This very brief protocol derives its name from administering large doses of benzodiazepines, usually Valium or Ativan, within the first twenty-four to forty-eight hours of withdrawal, after which the treatment is considered complete. An example of the approach would be to administer Valium 20 mg hourly, once the patient is entering into withdrawal, until a point of sedation, ataxia (mild balance impairment), or slurring of speech is reached. At this point, the benzodiazepine receptor would now be saturated with a long half-life benzodiazepine, which would therefore essentially function as a slow-release medication, covering the rest of withdrawal. Withdrawal would therefore be considered complete.

In all of these approaches, careful consideration must be given to the choice of benzodiazepine. A major difference between the two most commonly used, Valium and Ativan, is that Valium has a long elimination half-life. It also has an active metabolite which has a long half-life. This attribute means that the medication lasts much longer in the body, keeping the blood level more stable. These qualities are generally useful for withdrawal. Rivotril (clonazepam) and Librium (chlordiazepoxide) are two other examples of long-acting benzodiazepines that have been used for this purpose.

Long-acting benzodiazepines are not used in the elderly, or where any form of liver disease is present in the body. In such cases, the liver lacks the full capacity to metabolize or break down medication. This can cause an accumulation of the medication, causing toxicity, which in turn can lead to confusional states, oversedation, or falling. Ativan is a preferable option in these cases. It has a much lower likelihood of causing accumulation and subsequent toxicity.

Opiates

Increasingly, patients are being admitted for treatment of opiate dependence. There is little question that this is a significant growth area in addictions today. Opiate addiction may involve opiate prescription medications or heroin, which appears to be making a significant comeback. A rash of deaths from opiate overdose has been reported in both United States and Canada in recent months, particularly in middle-aged women, who may be mixing opiates with other sedative medications, leading to respiratory depression and death.

Many difficulties attend this dramatic rise. For one, the vast majority of these patients have acquired significant tolerance and their doses have escalated dramatically over the course of their addiction. Most have experienced withdrawal symptoms at some point, and as a result, they fear going through the process again. While some people describe opiate withdrawal as being like having a bad flu, most will say that it is not like any flu they have ever experienced before.

For another, it is often difficult for people to access appropriate withdrawal settings allowing them to get off these drugs, particularly the prescription medications (see below, Beyond Withdrawal, for more on this). They may have underlying pain issues which led them to use opiates in the first place, so part of their fear is related to how they will manage their pain once if they go off opiate medication.

Withdrawal. In the past, withdrawal from opiates generally involved use of nonopiate medications such as clonidine and a benzodiazepine, in addition to various other medications specifically targeted to one or two key withdrawal symptoms. For example, patients would be given clonidine .2 mg four times daily, in addition to Valium three or four times daily, with additional Maxeran or Gravol for nausea and vomiting and ibuprofen for muscle and joint aches. Despite this formidable combination of medications, patients withdrawing from opiates could be spotted immediately. They would be wrapped in a blanket, suffering hot and cold flashes, and holding a bucket or garbage pail to throw up in. They would often be irritable, angry, depressed, and extremely anxious. They did not sleep well, suffered muscle and joint aches, and appeared visibly uncomfortable. Their pupils were dilated. They were not happy campers.

Treatment. Withdrawal management improves dramatically with the use of methadone, which has a much higher level of patient acceptance than clonidine and Valium. A well-established protocol for management of heroin and prescription opiate withdrawal involves starting on methadone 10 mg four times daily. It is initially given in divided doses, to prevent the risk of overdosing with a single dose, thereby causing respiratory depression. This can be given for three days followed by a gradual tapering-off of 5 mg daily, until the tapering is complete and no more is given.

Another opiate used in detoxification — and one with less risk of toxicity — is Suboxone. This is a dual medication, containing a combination of naloxone and buprenorphine. Naloxone is an opiate *antagonist*, which means it blocks the effect of opiates. Buprenorphine is an *agonist*, which means that it allows the effect of opiates by activating the opiate receptor. Buprenorphine has what is called a high receptor affinity. It works by preferentially bumping the other opiates off the opiate receptor.

Naloxone is also used to treat patients who have overdosed on heroin or other opiates. It saves lives, although there are many stories of heroin addicts whose lives were saved when ambulance attendants administered naloxone, only to be met by angry heroin addicts in naloxone-induced opiate withdrawal who failed to appreciate that their life had been saved!

The interesting thing about Suboxone, a unique medication, is that it is administered as a tablet. It is designed to dissolve under the tongue, after which it is then absorbed into the body. In this form, the naloxone is not absorbed and has no effect. If an opiate addict were to take a Suboxone tablet, crush it, and dissolve it for injection, he would immediately go into withdrawal. The dual design of the tablet is meant to prevent such diversion and inappropriate use.

Buprenorphine is a *partial* agonist. Most opiates (including opiate prescription medications and heroin) are what are called *full* agonists. For purposes of discussion, let us describe a full agonist as having a 100 percent action and a partial agonist as having a 60 percent action. If a patient was admitted for detoxification, having used heroin in the parking lot just before walking in the door, she would already have a full agonist working on her opiate receptors; she would have no need for withdrawal management until the drug began to wear off and she went into acute withdrawal.

If we were to greet her at the door with a Suboxone tablet we would expect the following: she would put the tablet under her tongue, the tablet would dissolve, and she would absorb the buprenorphine, displacing the full-agonist heroin that she had used in the parking lot. This would result in precipitated withdrawal and a very unhappy patient!

Contrast this with a patient who entered treatment in acute opiate withdrawal—let's say, one who had used heroin in the parking lot the night before and now, the following morning, was in acute withdrawal. At this point, his opiate receptors would be running on empty. Administering the partial agonist would take him from 0 to 60 percent, and a marked reduction in withdrawal symptoms. We would now have a happy customer who was much more comfortable.

To avoid precipitated withdrawal, the challenge of when to start Suboxone is determined by an objective measurement of the patient's withdrawal state. To measure the extent of withdrawal, we commonly use COWS, the clinical opiate withdrawal scale. Generally speaking, once the opiate withdrawal score is over 10, patients are feeling quite uncomfortable and Suboxone treatment can be initiated. It is given in individualized doses, stabilizing the acute withdrawal; after that it is gradually tapered off over the following week to ten days.

Stimulants

Cocaine addiction leads to devastating consequences in a number of areas. With intoxication, medical risks are significant and can include seizures, hyperthermia, heart attacks, and death. In spite of this, no significant complications arise from withdrawal from these drugs. Even extremely heavy users are unlikely to have any serious medical concerns requiring treatment associated with withdrawal,. This is the case with cocaine and crack cocaine as well as methamphetamine. Classically, people withdrawing from these drugs struggle with fatigue, hypersomnia, and increased appetite — food is the withdrawal "medication" of choice!

Marijuana

A marijuana withdrawal syndrome has been described in the literature; however, no medical risks are associated with marijuana withdrawal.

Ecstasy/MDMA

It is rare to encounter people who use Ecstasy and MDMA daily for extended periods of time. More typically, these are drugs associated with bingeing, raves, and after-hour parties. There are no significant withdrawal risks associated with these drugs.

GHB

GHB is also commonly associated with bingeing, raves, and after-hour parties, but there is clearly a subgroup who engage in daily use of GHB over an extended period of time. These patients are at risk of developing withdrawal symptoms very much like those of alcohol withdrawal. These patients need to be closely managed and are generally treated in a manner similar to patients withdrawing from alcohol (Kamal et al. 2014).

Benzodiazepines

Benzodiazepine dependence is a relatively common presentation in withdrawal management units and residential treatment centres. People may have started using these drugs to treat anxiety or insomnia and then, long term, developed tolerance and dependence, as previously described. People may have acquired these medications from their own doctor, or alternatively from a variety of sources including other doctors, friends or families' medication, Internet sources, or the street. Benzodiazepines are frequently sought out by street drug users to assist with some of the side effects of stimulant drugs, for example coming down from stimulants. In British Columbia, some medical communities have access to PharmaNet, where prescription information is available online and prescribed medication can be confirmed for accuracy of reporting. It is important to check the patient's prescription bottles, to see if current medication supplies are consistent with the order on the label and date obtained.

Withdrawal can be very challenging, particularly when these medications were prescribed for treatment of anxiety or insomnia, because these symptoms are amplified in withdrawal. Ideally, benzodiazepines are tapered off in a very gradual fashion, over several months. This has been well described in the Ashton Manual (Ashton 2002). In residential treatment and withdrawal management settings, benzodiazepines are tapered off much more quickly, typically over a period of a few weeks; in addition, nonaddictive medications may be used to manage withdrawal symptoms.

Low-dose benzodiazepine withdrawal can generally be managed without switching medications. Moderate and higher doses of short-acting benzodiazepines will typically need to be converted to an equivalent dosage of a long-acting benzodiazepine such as diazepam (Valium) or clonazepam (Rivotril), which in turn can be tapered off. Equivalent dosage charts are readily available online.

The most challenging phase occurs toward the end of the taper, when withdrawal symptoms typically reach their peak. Benzodiazepine withdrawal symptoms can be quite variable and complex. They may also last for an extended period of time, often several months. Education and reassurance is an important feature of managing these patients.

Beyond Withdrawal: Treatment Options

Once a decision has been made to ask for help or seek assistance, and withdrawal is either complete or unnecessary, the next question is: what treatment option to pursue? Addiction disorders themselves vary significantly in severity, and treatment options also range widely—from making a contract to quit on one's own, to attending self-help groups, counselling or therapy, to the extreme of hospital admission or intensive residential treatment.

In any given community, a range of services is available for the treatment of addiction. However, in most geographic locations the demand for services is much greater than the supply, particularly on the more intensive end of the spectrum. This can be very frustrating for patients and families who decide to seek assistance, yet find that their setting of choice is not currently available. Wait lists are not uncommon, and waiting can be particularly problematic with addiction, where motivation to seek change is a moving target. A missed opportunity can be devastating.

That said, government-funded alcohol and drug treatment programs are available in most communities. Workers at these programs will be well aware of local resources for withdrawal, and outpatient or residential treatment. Family physicians are also generally well-informed regarding local resources and are good to consult about medical withdrawal issues or other drug- and alcohol-related medical complications.

Most communities have private therapists, several of whom may have specialized training in addiction. I would strongly recommend such a therapist. It is worth noting, however, that many otherwise excellent therapists do not have, specific training in alcohol and drug addiction.

In more urgent situations, local hospitals or emergency departments can provide assessment and referral. If withdrawal is not a major consideration, attendance at a local self-help group such as such as Rational Recovery©, Alcoholics Anonymous®, or Narcotics Anonymous can also be extremely helpful. Friends or family members of an alcoholic or drug addict can turn to specific twelve-step programs such as Al-Anon for support and guidance. For concerns more on the behavioural addiction side, government-funded sources of gambling treatment are available for individual counselling. A number of twelve-step programs are also available for addressing gambling disorders and sexually addictive behaviours. Many books have been written on these subjects; these can very usefully augment other types of therapy. Lastly, because addiction is often characterized by isolation, group therapy is a particularly helpful format for treatment.

The ASAM has created a publication to assist health professionals in appropriately matching severity of addiction to treatment settings, *ASAM Criteria: Treatment Criteria for Addictive, Substance-Related, and Co-occurring Conditions* (Mee-Lee 2013). (The document was previously entitled *ASAM PPC-2R: ASAM Patient Placement Criteria for the Treatment of Substance-Related Disorders*.) The ASAM has expanded the levels of service from five (for five different levels of addiction) to nine, utilizing the six dimensions of multidimensional assessment discussed previously, as follows.

Levels of Service in the ASAM PPC-2R

Level .5:   Early intervention
Level 1:   Outpatient services
Level 2:   Outpatient/partial hospitalization
Level 3:   Residential/inpatient
Level 4:   Medically managed intensive

Levels of Service in the Current ASAM Placement Criteria

Level .5:   Early intervention
Level 1:   Outpatient services
Level 2.1: Intensive outpatient services
Level 2.5: Partial hospitalization services
Level 3.1: Clinically managed intensity residential services
Level 3.3: Clinically managed population–specific high-intensity residential services
Level 3.5: Clinically managed high-intensity residential services
Level 3.7: Medically monitored intensive inpatient services
Level 4:   Medically managed intensive inpatient services

Outpatient treatment options range in intensity from Level 1 to Level 2.5, depending on need. Residential services also range in intensity, depending primarily on withdrawal risk, medical or psychiatric support/treatment required, motivation for change, relapse risk, and availability of community supports. A very helpful chart is available on pages 175 to 176 of the ASAM Criteria text (Mee-Lee 2013).

Early intervention may be indicated when individuals present with problems or issues potentially linked to alcohol and drug use, such as driving-related offences or various injuries or medical issues that have led to the need for medical care in a doctor's office or emergency room setting. Assessment of certain disruptive behaviours in various settings may turn up a possible problem with alcohol or drugs, and may suggest high-risk use of alcohol and drugs or an actual substance use disorder. In these situations, it is useful to determine the individual's motivation for making a change and to discuss positive steps or supports which may be helpful.

Outpatient services may be used as entry points for seeking treatment for addictions, or as a step down from more intensive treatment settings, such as residential treatment. They may use individual and/or group therapy for continuing counselling services. They may also be involved in assessment and referral to more intensive treatment settings. The effectiveness of both intensive outpatient programs (IOP) and residential treatment for addictions was confirmed in a very recent series of reviews in *Psychiatric Services'* Assessing the Evidence Base series. (McCarty et al. 2014; Reif et al. 2014).

Twelve-Step Approaches

Various self-help programs for substance abuse and behavioural addictions rely heavily on AA's famous twelve steps. These are listed in table 3.

I am repeatedly impressed by people who have been active participants in twelve-step programs over the long term. Many of my closest colleagues have had decades of sobriety and involvement with AA. The program encourages reaching out and helping others, a good foundation for continued psychological and spiritual growth. The beauty of the recovery process is that people do not have to struggle alone. Twelve-step meetings take place worldwide on a daily basis. To be a part of this international community is very reassuring for many.

Twelve-step language has been criticized by many people. The reader will immediately be impressed by the number of times that God is mentioned. This, combined with repeated declarations of AA's serenity prayer — "God, grant me the serenity to accept the things I cannot change, courage to change the things I can, and wisdom to know the difference" — often generates concerns for those who have no interest, or adverse reactions to, any form of religious exhortation.

Recently, a group of atheist alcoholics dealt with this concern by generating a version of the twelve-step program that does not mention the word "God" ("Atheist alcoholics seek to be well without 'God'" 2014). However, most twelve-step programs are actually nondenominational and do not make reference to any specific religion or belief system. Instead, they use terms like "God as we understand him" to describe the higher power, in an effort to apply broadly to a variety of religions. This flexibility is good news for some individuals, although it may be offensive (too liberal) for others with a more fundamentalist orientation.

Researchers and clinicians may take offence at AA's use of the term "powerless," since they feel that people suffering from addictions need to be empowered, not to have their feelings of being powerless further enhanced. However, the concept of powerlessness bears important witness to the personal history of addiction sufferers, who have been unable, many times before coming into treatment, to successfully control and manage their use of substances or addictive behaviours. Because these attempts have typically

Table 3
The Twelve Steps

---

1.   We admitted we were powerless over alcohol—that our lives had become unmanageable.

2.   Came to believe that a Power greater than ourselves could restore us to sanity.

3.   Made a decision to turn our will and our lives over to the care of God as we understood Him.

4.   Made a searching and fearless moral inventory of ourselves.

5.   Admitted to God, to ourselves and to another human being the exact nature of our wrongs.

6.   Were entirely ready to have God remove all these defects of character.

7.   Humbly asked Him to remove our shortcomings.

8.   Made a list of all persons we had harmed, and became willing to make amends to them all.

9.   Made direct amends to such people wherever possible, except when to do so would injure them or others.

10. Continued to take personal inventory and when we were wrong promptly admitted it.

11. Sought through prayer and meditation to improve our conscious contact with God, as we understood Him, praying only for knowledge of His will for us and the power to carry that out.

12. Having had a spiritual awakening as the result of these steps, we tried to carry this message to alcoholics, and to practice these principles in all our affairs.

---

not gone well, AA conceived of the necessity of finding a power greater than oneself—the famous "higher power" or "God as we understand him." This higher power can be interpreted various ways, but the essential meaning of the higher power is that it is something other than what has got you into your current predicament. "Your higher power can be many things, as long as you realize it's not you," they may say at meetings. Again, people with a well-established faith system may be offended by this concept, making it a barrier to engaging with the twelve-step program.

However, many of the twelve steps reinforce the idea of personal accountability for behaviour, particularly the effect that addiction has had on those closest to one. For example, Step 4 requires one to do a moral inventory, and Step 8 requires one to make appropriate amends to those one may have hurt. These steps, in my opinion, are really about personal growth and maturity. (See chapter 10 for a discussion of twelve-step facilitation therapy in the context of residential treatment.)

Other Self-Help Approaches

Twelve-step treatment has been a mainstay of addiction treatment for decades. However, several other common approaches may be used in place of, or in addition to, the twelve-step programs. Other well-known self-help approaches to addiction, including Rational Recovery® and SMART (an acronym for specific, measurable, assignable, realistic, and time-related), incorporate many practical approaches. They clearly distinguish themselves from twelve-step treatment programs by the absence of a spiritual component and do not generally see addiction as a disease.

Motivational Enhancement Therapy

Motivational enhancement therapy has been a very helpful treatment in motivating change in behaviour (Miller and Rollnick 2002). The treatment incorporates the stages of change model (Prochaska and DiClemente 1984), which distinguishes six stages that people go through as they consider making significant change, such as changing alcohol or drug consumption or other addictive behaviours. Prochaska and DiClemente argue for the need to consider the stage of change that a person is in, in order to assist them in moving them to the next stage. They suggest a variety of techniques for accomplishing this, discussed in detail in their book. The six stages of change are precontemplation, contemplation, determination, action, maintenance, and relapse.

Miller and Rollnick describe four general principles of motivational interviewing : express empathy, develop discrepancy between current behaviour and ideal goals and values; roll with resistance (as opposed to engaging in confrontation); and support self-efficacy. Proponents of this approach generally feel that it is much more supportive, collaborative, and less confrontational than the approach taken by traditional twelve-step programs.

Cognitive Behavioural Therapy (CBT)

Cognitive behavioural strategies are a foundation of outpatient and residential programs. A major focus of CBT is understanding triggers and cues, both internal and external, that cause cravings and the urge to return to addictive behaviours. Such cues may include uncomfortable emotional states such as anxiety, anger, resentment , or sadness. External stressors are often significant in early recovery. People and places associated with previous use can also be strong triggers. Understanding the triggers and cues, avoiding these when possible, and finding healthy alternative responses other than relapse are all important facets of CBT approaches. Many texts have been written describing cognitive behavioural approaches to addiction, including those by the renowned cognitive therapist Dr. Aaron Beck and colleagues (Beck et al. 1993). These concepts are also a core component of writings in the area of relapse prevention (Marlatt and Donovan 2005). These strategies have been used by members of Alcoholics Anonymous for years; they are reflected by the AA concern regarding "slippery people and places" and in the mnemonic for triggers, "HALT—hungry, angry, lonely, and tired."

Dialectical Behavioural Therapy (DBT)

DBT, initially developed by Dr. Marsha Linehan for treatment of borderline personality disorder, has also been extended for use in the treatment of addictions generally, and for patients with concurrent borderline personality disorder (Dimeff and Linehan 2008). A particular advantage of this approach is its focus on emotional regulation and stress management, which are well-known factors associated with relapse to alcohol and drugs and to other addictive behaviours. If stress and overwhelming emotion can be managed using these constructive approaches, relapse to alcohol and drugs and other addictive behaviours may be prevented.

DBT's specific behavioural targets for substance abuse include:

- Decreasing abuse of substances, including illicit drugs and legally prescribed drugs taken in a manner not prescribed.
- Alleviating physical discomfort associated with abstinence and/or withdrawal.
- Diminishing urges, cravings, and temptations to abuse.
- Avoiding opportunities and cues to abuse, for example by burning bridges to persons, places, and things associated with drug abuse and by destroying the telephone numbers of drug contacts, getting a new telephone number, and throwing away drug paraphernalia.
- Reducing behaviours conducive to drug abuse, such as momentarily giving up the goal to get off drugs and instead functioning as if the use of drugs cannot be avoided.

- Increasing community reinforcement of healthy behaviours, such as fostering the development of new friends, rekindling old friendships, pursuing social/vocational activities and seeking environments that support abstinence and punish behaviours related to drug abuse. (Dimeff and Linehan 2008)

DBT teaches four main skills that can readily be applied to addiction treatment: mindfulness, distress tolerance, emotional regulation, and interpersonal effectiveness. Acquisition of these skill sets can be extremely beneficial when applied to reducing relapse to alcohol and drugs or other addictive behaviours.

Harm Reduction and the Opioid Treatment Program (OTP)

Heroin addiction has been associated with many significant and devastating problems including contracting infectious diseases through injecting the drug, such as hepatitis C and HIV; elevated criminal behaviour; unstable housing and employment; violence; and significantly disrupted family life. Financial problems are often insurmountable. Many patients end up in prison, or dead from overdosing. Harm reduction, a very familiar term to substance abuse professionals and much of the lay population, aims to reduce these harmful consequences of addiction and improve addicts' quality of life, without necessarily reducing consumption of alcohol or drugs.

Harm reduction has a long history. Dr. Alan Marlatt provides a very interesting history of the practice of harm reduction, some of which is described below (Marlatt et al., 2012).

Holland has always been extremely progressive in the area of harm reduction, beginning with a government needle exchange in 1984, in which sterile syringes were provided to injection heroin addicts. The Dutch also actively prescribed methadone, in order to stabilize heroin addicts and reduce the harms associated with their addiction, including the transmission of HIV. By 2009, eighty-two countries all over the world had needle exchange programs and HIV transmission was significantly reduced.

The first government-sponsored needle exchange in North America was in Vancouver in 1989. By 2007, every province in Canada had a government-sponsored needle exchange program. Canada continues to be a leader in the area of harm reduction. Harm-reduction activities have included ongoing methadone and Suboxone maintenance programs, and research into assisted heroin treatments in which heroin addicts are provided pharmaceutical quality heroin to use in a supervised and safe setting.

The InSite program in Vancouver, started in 2003, is a legal, supervised injection site where heroin addicts can inject heroin in a supervised setting, preventing accidental death. This is the only such program in North America. Seven hundred people a day visit it. In 2009, a randomized controlled trial was initiated comparing a traditional continuum of care housing, where complete abstinence is required, to Housing First, where homeless people, typically with severe mental health and addiction issues, were housed with no obligation to be abstinent from alcohol and drugs. Recently reported results state that as a result of the program, over two thousand homeless Canadians found stable housing and that for every ten dollars spent there was a cost savings of twenty-two dollars (Goodman 2014). Over the last several years, several Canadian cities have developed managed alcohol programs, whereby previously homeless alcoholics are provided housing and given supervised alcohol. In one example, residents receive six ounces of white wine every ninety minutes, beginning at 8:00 in the morning continuing until 11:00 at night. The white wine replaces the very toxic forms of alcohol, including aftershave and shoe polish, that the homeless residents previously used.

Harm reduction clearly has very different goals from abstinence-based treatment. It is also generally recognized as dealing with a very different clientele. However, harm-reduction therapists are not opposed to abstinence as a goal, if this is the client's/patient's stated goal.

OTP programs are based on the harm-reduction philosophy of treatment. They involve management of opioid dependency using methadone or Suboxone/buprenorphine. Methadone and Suboxone substitution therapy for heroin addiction has been widely used since the early 1960s, when Dole and Nyswander published their initial paper in the *Journal of the American Medical Association* in 1965.

Opiate substitution therapies have been used for the treatment of heroin addiction for several decades. Heroin is a very short-acting drug in the opiate class. Individuals who are addicted to heroin require a repeated supply and their life typically revolves around maintaining their addiction. When they are unable to obtain money and drugs, they experience extremely uncomfortable withdrawal symptoms, creating a strong drive to maintain an ongoing supply. These patients reportedly do not do particularly well in abstinence-based treatments; other approaches need to be considered.

In substitution therapy, heroin is replaced with a prescribed opiate medication which remains in the body for a longer period of time and can be used once daily, or even less, thereby stabilizing the opiate system. The medication can be taken orally, eliminating the complications associated with injection drug use. When the opiate system is stabilized, drug-dependent individuals are able to focus on adaptive behaviours and goals rather than feeding their addiction. This approach has been highly successful and lifesaving for many individuals.

As research has progressed, there has been a much better awareness of optimal dosing, generally considered to be 60 mg or higher of methadone, significantly higher than in early years. Many physicians with an interest in addiction medicine have been actively involved in prescribing these medications for opiate-dependent patients in the community and in hospital settings. The ASAM recently published a detailed review of these practices (Fullerton et al. 2013). They find strong evidence for the effectiveness of methadone maintenance in retaining patients in treatment and reducing illicit opiate use. However, "evidence is less clear but suggestive that methadone maintenance treatment has a positive impact on mortality, illicit drug use (nonopioid), drug-related HIV risk behaviours, and criminal activity" (Brooks 2014).

Significantly, a large number of patients on substitution treatments continue to use illicit opiates. Many heroin addicts continue to abuse other drugs outside of the opiate class, which substitution therapy does not directly treat. As well, many opiate addicts have no interest in substitution therapies. Others have been on methadone for varying lengths of time and prefer not to be tied down to the program. All these patients may consider abstinence-based treatments as an alternative.

One area of contention between abstinence-based programs and harm-reduction clinicians has been the management of methadone in abstinence-based residential treatment programs. Methadone prescribers are often very pessimistic about the probability of opiate-dependent addicts remaining abstinent from opiates without long-term methadone. On the other hand, they see a potential benefit of having a patient attend residential treatment to abstain from nonopiate drugs or for treatment of behavioural addictions. Most residential treatment programs, being abstinence-based, do not support the continued use of any opiate, including methadone or Suboxone or buprenorphine in treatment. (This changed recently, when the Hazelden treatment facility in Minnesota decided to offer buprenorphine maintenance treatment for opiate addiction for the first time; Szalavitz 2012).

In such residential treatment programs, what happens when a user is admitted is that the methadone prescriber may advise against treatment, to avoid their patient coming off methadone. Alternatively, the patient may enter residential treatment with the onerous task of tapering off from methadone in order to achieve abstinence from opiates, often more rapidly than is generally recommended in community treatment settings. This inevitably leads to tension in the working relationship between the opiate-prescribing physician and the treatment program, rather than a cooperative approach.

In a disturbing recent trend, prescription opiate dependence has seen a dramatic escalation. There have been reports in Canada and the United States of greater numbers of deaths from accidental overdose of prescription opiates in the last several years. It is interesting to consider whether the current patients, many of whom become addicted to prescription opiates, will have a different response to various treatments available than the more traditional heroin addicts.

Case Study

FRED

Fred, 27, lives with his parents in a major urban centre. He has been in a relationship with a woman for five years. He has not been married and has no children. He is a business owner and entrepreneur. Fred was admitted to Edgewood following an intervention organized by his family, for treatment of benzodiazepine and opiate dependence. At the time of admission, he was on large doses of benzodiazepines and opiates.

Fred was initially prescribed Imovane for insomnia at the age of 17, typically taking three tablets nightly. By the age of 21, he was receiving benzodiazepines for treatment of anxiety. This was prescribed by his psychiatrist. He developed significant tolerance and dependence, and took any combination of clonazepam, diazepam, alprazolam, and lorazepam in very large doses. He acquired numerous tablets of diazepam when travelling abroad, where prescriptions are not required. Two different doctors prescribed three other benzodiazepines for him. He suffered a seizure one year ago, when he tried to taper his use.

He has also been addicted to prescription opiates for the last few years, taking over 1000 mg daily of OxyContin. In addition, his own doctor had prescribed Tylenol 3. He had been diagnosed with attention deficit disorder (ADD) in elementary school and lately had begun taking prescription stimulants for energy. He had also been using marijuana on a nightly basis since junior high school, and had significant problems with gambling and sexually addictive behaviours.

Fred stated that he had always had significant behaviour problems, beginning in elementary school. He did not do well with authority figures. He became involved in theft and had sold drugs at school. At one point, he did extremely well in business, however this later fell apart leading to significant stress, and increased anxiety and insomnia. He had no history of suicidal thoughts or attempts. He had tried a number of antidepressants but never gave them a reasonable try. He stated that there was a family history of addiction on both sides of the family.

Fred clearly required detoxification from two different classes of medications. While opiate withdrawal is extremely uncomfortable, it is not dangerous or life-threatening; benzodiazepine withdrawal management was the priority. As Fred is a young man, and in the absence of any known liver problems, he underwent detoxification using diazepam, a long-acting benzodiazepine.

Regardless of how much benzodiazepines a patient may be taking, Edgewood's ceiling starting dose is 20 mg four times daily, with a possible additional 20 mg during the night if needed. This would be tapered gradually over the following 30 days according to a scheduled withdrawal protocol. The rate of tapering would need to be much slower on an outpatient basis.

Opiate withdrawal was managed with Suboxone, instituted on the second full day in treatment. Caution was exercised when combining the two sedative medications, because they could have an additive effect on respiratory function. Fred was given an initial dose of 4 mg of Suboxone. This was repeated four hours later as his withdrawal symptoms remained moderately severe. The following day, he required 12 mg which was his maximum dose. The Suboxone was also tapered over approximately the next ten days. Not surprisingly, Fred experienced significant difficulties with anxiety and insomnia as the tapering treatment progressed. This was managed with nonaddictive medications, specifically Gabapentin 300 mg four times daily, increased gradually to 600 mg four times daily over the next several days. Anxiety and sleep issues improved considerably. Trazodone 50 to100 mg was also added to help him sleep. Trazodone has a rare but very important potential side effect in men: priapism, which is a sustained erection requiring surgery. It is important to explain this potential side effect for the purposes of informed consent. Over the following several weeks, his Gabapentin dosage was reduced; however, he remained on 600 mg at bedtime only, as well as on Trazodone 100 mg HS. Gabapentin and Trazodone, both nonaddictive medications, were used off indication; that is, they were not specifically approved and marketed for this purpose. This was explained to Fred.

Chapter 8

Hot Topics

Opiate Issues

Probably more than any other area of addiction medicine, the treatment of opiate dependence tends to polarize treatment providers. I recall presenting a talk at a major addiction conference in Canada that had nothing to do with opiates or methadone maintenance. Following my presentation, the first question from the audience was "as an abstinence-based treatment program, why are you discriminating against our methadone patients by not allowing them to enter your treatment programs?" Often, treatment providers are caught between immediate goals of detoxification followed by abstinence, on the one hand, and opioid replacement therapy with methadone or buprenorphine, with or without an ultimate long-term goal of abstinence on the other.

This controversy is likely to continue, because opiate dependence treatment is increasingly a priority. By 2010, drug overdose deaths increased for the eleventh consecutive year (Paulozzi et al. 2012). Overdose deaths involving opioid analgesics showed a similar increase. Starting with 4,030 deaths in 1999, the number of these deaths increased to 15,597 in 2009 and 16,651 in 2010. Nearly 60 percent of drug overdose deaths involved pharmaceutical drugs, and opioid analgesics were involved in about three of every four pharmaceutical overdose deaths, confirming the predominant role opioid analgesics have played in drug overdose deaths in this period.

A posting on the Office of National Drug Control Policy blog on February 11, 2014 stated:

The abuse of opioids—a group of drugs that includes heroin and prescription painkillers—is having a devastating impact on public health and safety in communities across the nation. . . . More Americans are using and dying from prescription painkillers than from heroin. According to the Centres for Disease Control and Prevention (CDC), we've seen roughly a 20 percent increase in overdose deaths involving prescription painkillers since 2006. In 2010, there were over 16,000 drug poisoning deaths involving prescription painkillers. There were about 3,000 drug poisoning deaths involving heroin that same year. (Hardesty 2014).

The report also noted that methadone accounts for nearly one in three prescription painkiller overdose deaths in the United States, even though only 2 percent of prescriptions for opiate painkillers are for this drug. (It is extremely important to note that the majority of the deaths related to methadone patients are being treated for pain, *not* methadone maintenance for addiction.)

In general, a similar trend is being observed in Canada. In 2013, British Columbia's provincial health officer, in collaboration with other health officials and the police, posted an alert about potential overdoses associated with illicit use of the drug fentanyl ("Opioid Overdose in BC" 2013). A synthetic opioid many times more potent than morphine, fentanyl was being marketed at the street level as OxyContin, when that drug was removed due to high rates of abuse (see chapter 2, Availability). Because fentanyl is much more powerful than other opioids, the risk of an accidental overdose is obviously much higher. Fentanyl has also recently been found in contaminated heroin in the United States, leading to numerous accidental deaths (SAMHSA 2014.)

Further research into the area of prescription opiate dependence, as opposed to heroin dependence, is essential in order to prescribe the most appropriate treatment for given patients. In light of this escalating need to find ways of dealing with the prescription opiate addiction epidemic, several interesting observations come to mind.

Shift from Heroin to Prescription Opiates

Opiate addiction has changed over the last few decades. Heroin used to be the opiate of choice for users, but now it seems that prescription opiates have taken heroin's place. Several questions arise as to whether previous data specific to heroin are appropriately transferable to prescription opiate dependence. Specifically, should a goal of abstinence be considered, with or without the addition of naltrexone (which would prevent users from getting high)? Should prescription opiate addicts be treated with traditional opiate replacement therapy? Is there some means to identify the best treatment option for a specific individual?

Recovery from Opiate Addiction without Treatment

Some fascinating research describes heroin addicts who were able to enter into longer-term abstinence without treatment of any type, and re-enter a more normal life (Biernacki 1986). Biernacki's sample of 101 patients had been addicted to heroin for at least one year and were now, subsequently, free of addiction for at least two years. The findings in his research are described under four main headings: resolving to stop, breaking away from addiction, staying abstinent, and becoming and being "ordinary" ("Stopping Heroin Use without Treatment" n.d.)

Vietnam Veterans and Opiate Addiction

Up to 20 percent of soldiers in Vietnam became addicted to heroin during the course of their active military involvement, yet only a very small percentage of these veterans remained addicted after returning to the United States (Robins 1993). Only 12 percent of those addicted in Vietnam had been addicted at any time in the three years since their return. Other findings in this study were that heroin was highly accessible and cheap, and that marijuana use was also highly prevalent—"close to 80 percent of enlisted men [were] using marijuana." The strongest predictors of becoming addicted to opiates were found to be early behaviour problems and drug use prior to joining the military, rather than exposure to traumatic events while serving.

Opiate Addiction and the Environment

The role of the environment in perpetuating addictive behaviour has been explored in a fascinating Canadian study, "Addiction: The View from Rat Park" (Alexander n.d.). The addictive behaviour of the opiate-addicted rats in that study, with animals tightly enclosed in a cage, has been reproduced in various studies. When similarly addicted rats were placed in a spacious, rat-friendly environment, with the same opportunity to pursue water containing opiates, they declined to do so. They failed to exhibit the addictive behaviour. The author's conclusion, as reported to the Canadian Senate in 2001, was: "severely distressed animals, like severely distressed people, will relieve their distress pharmacologically if they can."

Alleged Poor Outcomes of Abstinence-Based Treatment

Numerous studies and reports have made reference to the poor outcomes associated with abstinence-based treatment in the treatment of heroin-dependent subjects. Yet, at the same time, most would see successful long-term abstinence as the most desirable endpoint of treatment. The National Treatment Outcome Research Study (NTORS) looked at five-year outcomes following treatment of various types in the UK (Gossop et al. 2001). Of the 650-patient sample, 13 percent were inpatients; 26 percent were rehabilitation patients; 18 percent were on methadone reduction; and 43 percent were on methadone maintenance. NTORS was able to do a four- or five-year follow-up of 76 percent of the original 650 clients in treatment.

The most common diagnosis was long-term opiate dependence (usually heroin) of an extensive and chronic nature. The average duration of heroin use was nine years, and almost two-thirds of the sample were injecting drugs prior to intake. Importantly, the clients in the residential programs had more serious problems than those in the outpatient programs. In spite of this, 38 percent of the residential clients were abstinent from all six of illicit target drugs at four to five years. The percentage of residential clients who were abstinent from illicit opiates — the main problem drugs at intake — increased from 19 percent at intake to 47 percent after five years. For the methadone clients, more than a third were abstinent from illicit opiates at four to five years. Daily use of opiates among the residential clients had fallen from 51 percent for treatment to 18 percent at four to five years. Eighty percent of the methadone clients were regularly using heroin. After one year, this fell to 50 percent and decreased further to 42 percent at the four- to five-year follow-up. Regular use of nonprescribed methadone was reported by thirty-one percent of these clients at intake. This dropped by nearly two-thirds, to 11 percent at one year.

Similar results were noted in an Irish study (Smyth et al. 2005), in which 23 percent of heroin addicts admitted for detoxification followed by inpatient services remained abstinent at two to three years after inpatient treatment. Abstinence was significantly associated with completion of the six-week inpatient treatment program and attendance at outpatient aftercare. These studies challenge the common allegation that abstinence is not possible for opiate and heroin addicts.

Treatment of Health Care Professionals

A significant number of health professionals are addicted to opiates. Many treatment programs are available for them. Almost all choose abstinence-based programs, supposedly to avoid the cognitive side effects associated with opiate replacement therapies, which they believe could affect their decision-making capacity and generate a risk to patients under their care. Health care professionals have among the highest rates of prolonged abstinence success, approaching 80 percent over five years. This leads one to question what other groups of patients could have similar success with abstinence, and what features of treatment could lead to these levels of success.

These issues are explored further in an article reviewing the concerns related to opiate replacement therapy for health care professionals; the article also explores the position that various professional health programs have taken on the subject (Fiscella 2012). The author's experience was that many state health programs were reluctant to disclose their specific policies in this area.

Opiate Replacement Therapies

Opiate replacement therapies have very clearly demonstrated, important benefits including improved retention, reduced use of illicit opiates, improved quality of life, and reduction of risks associated with intravenous drug use. A number of patients in opiate replacement therapy do not like being tied down to their treatment, or expressed concern about side effects associated with treatment. Many patients in opiate replacement treatment continue to abuse or become dependent on other classes of drugs; however, many eventually choose a goal of abstinence, with the delayed challenge of ultimately getting off opiates.

Medication Treatments
for Substance Dependence

Smoking Cessation

Medications to assist with smoking cessation have been available for several years. To assist with withdrawal from smoking — and ideally to promote abstinence — nicotine is available in lozenges, gum, and patches. Bupropion (marketed as Zyban for smoking cessation) has been used for several years to assist with smoking cessation. This medication doubles the chance of quitting smoking successfully after three months and has a 1.5 times higher abstinence rate than a placebo one year after treatment. Its use is complicated by the fact that it is an antidepressant (also marketed as Wellbutrin) so other considerations are important, particularly any possibility of bipolar disorder.

Varenicline (marketed Champix in Canada and as Chantix in the United States) is a nicotinic receptor partial agonist on the nicotinic receptor in the brain, where nicotine normally exerts its action. This means that it will activate nicotinic receptor in a manner similar to nicotine, but to a lesser extent (see the similar discussion of buprenorphine in chapter 3, Opiates). The drug significantly reduces withdrawal issues commonly noted with discontinuing nicotine, such as cravings, increased appetite, and irritability. It has been found to be significantly more effective than a placebo. A small percentage of people who have used it experienced significant depression and suicidal ideation, so people on this drug need to be closely monitored, and be informed of this risk. It is generally taken for twelve weeks.

Alcohol Dependence

The role of medication in the treatment of alcohol dependence has been extensively reviewed in a recent article (Robinson 2014). A few of the options are highlighted here.

Antabuse has been available for many years. It blocks one of the enzymes (aldehyde dehydrogenase) that is required for complete metabolism of alcohol. If someone drinks alcohol while taking Antabuse, elevated levels of an intermediate product called acetaldehyde are formed. This causes very uncomfortable side effects that therefore have a deterrent effect on drinking. Antabuse can be taken daily for extended periods of time, or alternatively, it may be used in the short term for high-risk relapse scenarios such as anniversaries related to loss and grief, weddings, or Christmas and New Year's. Obviously, it only works if someone is taking it, so compliance is therefore a very important issue. It is best used for prevention of impulsive drinking and will not stop premeditated calculated relapses.

It is important to be cautious. Some skin products contain alcohol, which can be absorbed into the body; such unexpected ingested sources of alcohol can trigger a reaction. Of interest, I have met many alcoholics who relapsed, admitting to experimenting with gradually increasing amounts of alcohol while continuing to take Antabuse, to see how much they could get away with — even under the supervision of a spouse or partner.

Naltrexone, marketed as Revia, has also been available for several years. It is a well-known opiate receptor antagonist, used to reduce the frequency and severity of relapses to drinking. There is also evidence that naltrexone helps reduce heavy drinking when people who are taking the drug also continue to drink.

Acamprosate, marketed as Campral, appears to have an action on the GABA/glutamate systems:

It appears to be an effective and safe treatment strategy for supporting continuous abstinence after detoxification in alcohol-dependent patients. Although . . . treatment effects appear to be rather moderate in their magnitude, they should be valued against the background of the relapsing nature of alcoholism and the limited therapeutic options currently available for its treatment. (Rösner et al. 2011)

Both naltrexone and acamprosate, while being supported in research, have received limited enthusiasm from clinicians in the field. A variety of factors probably account for this, including skepticism regarding using a drug to treat addiction; limited benefits; cost; anticipated compliance problems; and the belief that medications should not be required if people are working an appropriate recovery program.

Topirimate, marketed as Topamax, has been studied for its potential benefit in preventing relapse in alcoholics. Initial research looks promising although side effects from this medication, particularly in the area of cognition, can lead to reservations in using it for this purpose (Sommer et al. 2013; Thompson et al. 2000).

Stimulant Dependence

Considerable research has been undertaken in the quest to find a medication or medications that may be helpful in reducing relapse to cocaine, crack cocaine, and methamphetamine. At this time, no available medications clearly reduce relapse rates for these drugs, although several medications, under study by the National Institute of Drug Abuse (NIDA) and others, continue to be potential candidates (National Institute on Drug Abuse 2013).

Medical Marijuana

Marijuana is a plant product which contains 489 distinct compounds in eighteen chemical classes. Marijuana is chiefly associated with tetrahydrocannabinol (THC), its single most active ingredient, but in fact there are over seventy different cannabinoids in marijuana.

Drugs exert their action by attaching to a receptor in the brain, where a response is triggered. Several years ago, it was discovered that our bodies contain cannabinoid receptors, which work in a similar way to opiate receptors (see chapter 3, Opiates); when activated, these receptors produce the high sought by the user. It turns out that our body has a similar arrangement with cannabinoids. Cannabinoid receptors are located in the brain, along the spinal column, and widely distributed in most organs in the body. They can be activated through external consumption of cannabinoids such as marijuana—or with cannabinoids our own bodies make. Of these, the two best-known are Anandamide and 2-Arachidoylglycerol (2-AG). We have two different types of cannabinoid receptors, labelled CB1 and CB2. The CB1 receptors tend to be located in the brain whereas CB2 receptors tend to be located elsewhere in the body. We might wonder why our bodies have cannabinoid receptors in the first place, and what the functions of this cannabinoid system are—presumably, their primary function was not to get high on marijuana! Actually, researchers have discovered that the cannabinoid system functions in a variety of areas including memory, energy balance, metabolism and—not surprisingly—appetite. Think marijuana munchies! Additionally, the system appears to have an important function in the immune system and the experience of pain/analgesia. It also appears to have a role in sleep, and probably with female reproductive issues (Health Canada 2013).

When one considers the many areas of function of the cannabinoid system, one can easily speculate that there could be ways in which the cannabinoid system could be modulated to potentially improve function and assist with disease. There could also be disorders of the cannabinoid system. Alternatively, external use of cannabinoids could disrupt the normal function of the cannabinoid system, generating problems or disorders.

Medical Marijuana in Canada

In Canada, physicians were originally able to prescribe marijuana to patients under certain criteria, according to Health Canada's Marihuana Medical

Access Regulations, which were in effect prior to March 31, 2014 (Health Canada 2014). Table 4 lists these criteria.

As of March 1, 2014 the program's name changed to Marihuana for Medical Purposes Regulations (see Health Canada 2014 for more information).

Health Canada had previously identified a number of specific categories of treatment indications. Under the new regulations, a document signed by a practising physician or licensed health care practitioner (such as a nurse practitioner) can be directly submitted to a licensed producer who will then provide medical marijuana. This has opened up the indications considerably. (For a further discussion of the current situation, see Illegality of Marijuana, below.)

Medical marijuana comes in a variety of forms:

- *Smoked marijuana* which contains numerous compounds and over seventy different cannabinoids.
- *Sativex*, a mouth spray containing THC and cannabidiol. Cannabidiol is the second most common cannabinoid found in smoked marijuana. It does not cause euphoria and may be responsible for some of the treatment benefits in various conditions.
- *Marinol/dronabinol*, a synthetic THC.
- *Nabilone/ cesamet*, a synthetic cannabinoid, not THC. There are only rare reports of addiction associated with its use.

Cannabinoids are now being investigated by researchers for treatment of various medical disorders. Their antineoplastic properties may help fight cancer, and they have anticonvulsant properties. They may help chronic pain, and can help to reduce the intraocular pressure caused by glaucoma.

Table 4
Canadian Medical Marijuana Criteria

	Criteria
Category 1	Any symptom treated as part of compassionate end-of-life care
	Symptoms related to specific medical conditions, namely: • severe pain and/or persistent muscle spasms from multiple sclerosis • severe pain and/or persistent muscle spasms from a spinal cord injury • severe pain and/or persistent muscle spasms from a spinal cord disease • severe pain, cachexia (muscle wasting), anorexia, weight loss and/or severe nausea from cancer or HIV/AIDS infection • severe pain from severe forms of arthritis • seizures from epilepsy
Category 2	A debilitating symptom that is associated with a medical condition or with the medical treatment of that condition, other than those described in Category 1

They can also help sleep disorders, and are already being used to assist with sleep disturbances caused by PTSD. There is interest in cannabidiol in the treatment of anxiety and schizophrenia. This is of particular interest, as this cannabinoid is unlikely to cause addiction. Cannabinoids may also have a neuroprotective effect, which may be beneficial for dementia and inflammatory bowel disease. There is an excellent, up-to-date review of the research on the Health Canada website by a group of international experts for those wishing to pursue this further (Health Canada 2013).

Medical Marijuana Issues

As marijuana becomes more readily available through medical marijuana programs and through newly sanctioned recreational use in the United States, new concerns have emerged that need to be addressed.

Impairment. Marijuana intoxication causes a level of impairment, clearly a concern for motor vehicle drivers and in employment situations involving safety sensitivity. With alcohol, a breathalyzer test can be performed and well-established standards are in place to measure impairment. By contrast, currently used drug tests for detection of THC will generate a positive result, demonstrating that someone has used marijuana — but these tests do not demonstrate impairment. If someone used marijuana on Saturday and Sunday, and showed up to work on Monday morning, their screening test would probably be positive even though they had not used for many hours and were not now high. This is a current area of research and needs to be sorted out in the near future.

Increased use by adolescents. A major concern related to increased availability of marijuana is increased access to and use by adolescents, whose brains continue to develop into their early twenties. Several research studies have signalled that this may be a problem; however, research findings are inconsistent (Volkow, Baler et al. 2014).

Illegality of marijuana. Marijuana has been used for numerous medicinal purposes for hundreds of years in various regions of the world. In traditional Chinese medicine, it is one of the fifty fundamental herbs. In spite of this, marijuana is currently classified as an illegal drug.

In the United States, marijuana is a Schedule 1 substance, meaning that "growing, distribution or possession [of it] is a federal crime regardless of state law." In the last several years a number of American states, starting with California, have legalized marijuana for medicinal purposes. At the time of writing, twenty states and the District of Columbia have legalized medical marijuana. Colorado and the state of Washington have legalized the recreational use of cannabis as well. In spite of the fact that many states have legalized medical marijuana, it remains illegal by federal law, although recent federal changes have been instituted to move in the direction of accommodating state law with respect to medical marijuana.

In Canada, the Marihuana Medical Access Program was introduced in 2001 (Health Canada 2014). At that time, fewer than 100 people were authorized to possess marijuana for medical purposes, and "over the years that number has grown to close to 40,000" (Health Canada's New Rules" 2014). In the centralized Canadian program, there were essentially three ways to obtain marijuana for medical purposes: growing your own, delegating a grower, or receiving a supply from Health Canada. Applications for the program, based on medical eligibility and accompanied by physician's letter, would be sent to Health Canada.

In early 2014, Health Canada was in the middle of a major change in the program. Initially, they decided to ban individuals from growing their own marijuana or delegating another party to grow for them, and excluded themselves as suppliers of marijuana for the program. Instead, in an attempt to make marijuana like "other prescription narcotics," a group of designated suppliers, growing commercial marijuana, would make it available by physician prescription. This led to considerable objection and a subsequent legal appeal. New laws that were to go into effect on April 1, 2014 have been delayed pending the outcome of the court decision.

Concerns included the increased cost of obtaining marijuana through the new program, probable limitations in accessing physicians who were willing to participate in the program, and some loss of autonomy. Law enforcement officials and fire department officials continued to have major concerns about growing marijuana at home due to the fire risk associated with electrical issues, and criminal enforcement issues related to growing drugs.

Concerns often raised were risk of addiction, the role of physicians in the medical marijuana program, and the role of patients in the program.

Risk of addiction. On the addiction side, addiction specialists continue to be concerned about the potential risk of people becoming addicted to marijuana. Current estimates are that approximately 10 percent of regular users would become marijuana dependent. Because of the laxity of the medical marijuana program, many have felt that people would use it for addiction purposes rather than for legitimate medical problems. In my clinical practice, I have clearly seen it used as a mechanism to continue to supply marijuana for a marijuana-dependent individual, and also to cover for those who were selling marijuana. This is not to say many individuals did not use it appropriately.

The role of physicians in the medical marijuana program.

Almost without exception, every major medical body has voiced its opposition, either to the program itself, or the role of the physician described in the program. Common concerns include a lack of training or education involved with medical marijuana, the absence of quality control of the product itself in contrast to pharmaceutical substances, the absence of a process similar to that which is expected of any other new drug entering the marketplace, and a limited set of clinical trials documenting the efficacy of medical marijuana for the conditions for which it is being promoted. Most physicians were not familiar with dosing and data were generally limited in this regard.

The role of patients. Many patients were concerned that the new process would lead to dramatically elevated prices, and therefore potentially limit their access to their desired treatment. They might also be using a particular strain or product that is currently helpful, and not want to change it.

Occupational Addiction

The last several years has seen a dramatic increase in interest in occupational addiction medicine. This is not surprising, since addiction and mental illness are leading causes of disability worldwide. According to the Canadian Centre for Substance Abuse, statistics from 2002 data (the most recent available) show that costs attributable to substance abuse are approximately $40 billion (Richter et al. 2002). Productivity loss accounts for $24 billion. Tobacco and alcohol account for 80 percent while illegal drugs account for approximately 20 percent of these figures. Addiction in the workplace causes increases in rates of premature death and fatal accidents, injuries, absenteeism, loss of productivity, lateness, theft, and extensive medical, rehabilitation, and employee assistant program costs. It also reduces morale and causes relationship strain among coworkers, leading to higher staff turnover, the need for training new employees, and instituting various disciplinary procedures, as well as the cost of drug testing. Increasing expectations have been placed on employers to provide a safe workplace setting. The concept of safety has extended to include a psychologically safe environment as well as a physical one. Employers must meet the requirements of human rights legislation, union contracts, legal obligations, and known industry standards in consideration of alcohol and drug policies in the workplace.

Under Canadian human rights legislation, alcohol and/or drug dependence is considered a disability and employers are not allowed to discriminate on the basis of the presence of a medical disability, any more than they could discriminate on the basis of heart disease or musculoskeletal injury. There is thus a legal duty to accommodate an employee and work around their disability in a reasonable manner unless to do so can be demonstrated to cause undue hardship. Detailed descriptions of both duty to accommodate and undue hardship are provided in the legislation (Canadian Human Rights Commission 2009).

The transition from DSM-IV-TR to DSM-5 has muddied the water considerably in this area. Workplace protocols typically responded to abuse and dependence differently. Workplace policies and procedures were consistent with the language of DSM-IV-TR. Human rights legislation recognized dependence as a disease, but abuse was not considered a disease and complaints were thus not supported. There is no clearly established relationship between the language of DSM-IV-TR and DSM-5 with regard to addiction, leaving the occupational field of addiction with considerable ambiguity. This will likely need to be resolved through the courts in the future.

Because of the increased focus on and escalating responsibility for employees who have addiction issues, workplace drug testing has become an increasingly common requirement. Pre-employment testing for the purpose of identifying drug users is common practice. Random drug testing of employees working in safety-sensitive positions, in which impairment could endanger the employee or other employees, is an increasingly common practice where employers and unions have agreed to it. In two high-profile Canadian legal cases, employers unilaterally instituted random screening for detection of alcohol and drugs for employees in safety-sensitive positions. One company instituted random breathalyzer testing for alcohol in its safety-sensitive positions. This practice was struck down by the courts. The other instituted random drug screening for its safety-sensitive employees. Courts did not support this practice either. This is clearly an evolving area (Smith 2014; Supreme Court of Canada 2013).

Testing is also commonly used for postaccident and reasonable suspicion, based on an employee's behaviour. Employees in safety-sensitive positions, returning to work after addiction treatment, are also required to commit to random drug testing as well as various other components of a return-to-work agreement. This agreement will generally consist of follow-up appointments with an addiction specialist, random drug testing, and probable involvement in twelve-step meetings such as Alcoholics Anonymous or Narcotics Anonymous. These contracts have been shown to increase long-term abstinence and therefore provide a safer workplace.

Case Study: Gord

Gord, fifty-four, was admitted for treatment of alcohol and marijuana dependence. Gord was born and raised in a small community on Vancouver Island. He was married for twelve years before his divorce ten years ago. He had two sons in their late teens who were now living with their mother. He maintained regular contact with them. Gord had been employed by his current employer in the forestry industry for fifteen years. He worked dayshift and was currently single.

Gord described a reasonably positive upbringing. His father was involved in logging and his mother was a homemaker, who looked after him, his older brother, and younger sister. He described some tendency toward verbal abuse in the family. He was involved in sports in high school and later played drums in a band. He was not aware of any sexual abuse. He stated that he had lost several friends, for various reasons, and was also in a serious motor vehicle accident years ago with his wife. The accident was not associated with his drinking, and was described as the fault of the other party; both members of the other party were killed. He recalls having some time-limited PTSD symptoms; these did not remain and were not present currently.

Gord described a maternal uncle, his maternal grandfather, and his brother as alcoholics. His brother was currently doing much better. He believed that his mother's side of the family, including his mother, suffered from depression and anxiety.

Gord stated that he had been a daily drinker for the last five years. He typically drank after supper, as he was concerned about his blood sugar, being a diabetic. After eating, he would consume as many as twelve beers and thirteen ounces of hard liquor. This had been his pattern for at least the last couple of years. He described a gradual escalation of his drinking, particularly after his separation and divorce several years ago. Significantly, he noted that his wife had been concerned about his drinking, which was allegedly more problematic on weekends prior to separating.

Gord stated that his addiction issues came to the attention of his employer when he accidentally pulled out a marijuana joint rather than a roll-your-own cigarette. This led to an honest discussion with his immediate supervisor regarding his addiction to alcohol and marijuana. His employer arranged for him to get residential treatment and he also signed a contract for return to work, monitoring, and aftercare programs.

This was apparently his first work-related incident, and he denied any problems with absenteeism. He stated that he did not drink in the morning or during the day. Similarly, he denied using marijuana at work. He described being in a safety-sensitive position at work. He had regularly been having blackouts. He had a ninety-day suspension following an impaired driving charge six years ago. He denied any twenty-four–hour suspensions or incarcerations related to drinking. He stated that he did not get into fights or physical altercations.

Gord began using marijuana at the age of twelve. He was using daily by the age of thirteen, with a pattern of recurrent use throughout the day. He had essentially continued daily marijuana use ever since, although he apparently had restricted his daytime use in the last five or six years. He had used cocaine and Ecstasy very infrequently over the years, and used LSD fairly regularly in high school. He had not abused prescription medications. He did not endorse symptoms of pathological gambling or sexually addictive behaviours.

Following his separation, Gord reportedly saw a psychiatrist once for assessment of depressive symptoms. He had been on antidepressants briefly at this time but felt they were not effective. Then, one year previously, he had gone to his doctor with concerns about depression and was started on Cipralex. He was currently taking 30 mg daily. He did not notice any improvement with the antidepressant. He was also taking appropriate medications for Type 2 diabetes, hypertension, and elevated cholesterol. He lost seventy-five or eighty pounds after being diagnosed with diabetes.

Gord attributed his depressive symptoms primarily to loneliness. He tended to feel better at work when he was distracted, he said, and in a more social setting. He had become increasingly isolated as his alcohol dependence progressed. In terms of anxiety, he described fairly typical generalized anxiety and social anxiety. He remembered being bullied and teased throughout his school years. He described having a difficult time in school and had to repeat Grades 6 and 7. He subsequently went into a more technical stream and managed to get his Grade 12. He believed he saw a specialist for educational difficulties but had not gone on medications. He wondered if he had attention deficit hyperactivity disorder (ADHD). There was no history of suicide attempts. He did have fleeting suicidal thoughts following the separation, and got rid of his guns at the time to avoid any impulsive actions while intoxicated.

Chapter 9

Concurrent Disorders

Concurrent disorders have attracted considerable interest in the last couple of decades, in addiction medicine and elsewhere. In addiction medicine, the term refers to the presence of a substance use disorder in conjunction with at least one identified DSM-5 psychiatric disorder. Often, more than one psychiatric disorder co-occurs with a substance use disorder.

It is estimated that at least one-quarter of patients suffering from major depression and anxiety disorders have a comorbid (concurrent) substance abuse disorder. Patients with more severe mental illnesses such as bipolar disorder and schizophrenia have considerably higher rates. Individuals with ADHD also have higher rates of addiction to various substances. A recent study looking at the comorbidity of severe psychotic disorders with measures of substance abuse found an approximate fourfold risk of smoking, heavy alcohol use, heavy marijuana use, and recreational drug use (Hartz et al. 2014). If we were also to include cigarette smoking and nicotine dependence, the rates would approach 80 or 90 percent.

In order to treat concurrent disorders appropriately, it is very important for practitioners to have the appropriate tools and training. They must identify the disorders, and implement a comprehensive treatment plan consistent with best practice guidelines for both disorders. This can be challenging at the best of times, for several reasons. Significantly, there are very well-developed best practice guidelines for individual psychiatric disorders, but specific research in the area of concurrent disorders has been extremely limited. Previous research into specific psychiatric disorders has excluded patients with substance use disorders. As well, behavioural addictions or the use of alcohol and drugs may mask or mimic various psychiatric disorders. Some common clinical challenges are discussed in the sections below.

Treatment Centre Challenges

In 2001, the ASAM identified treatment centres providing concurrent psychiatric care according to three levels (Mee-Lee 2001, 2013). The first was *basic residential treatment* with no additional psychiatric care. (These days, all treatment settings should generally be capable of providing some level of psychiatric assessment and treatment as a minimal standard.) The second level was *dual-diagnosis capable* with access to psychiatric assessment and treatment of mild to possibly moderate levels of psychiatric disorder, with the primary focus being the treatment of addiction. The third level of care identified was a true *dual-disorder program* with specific, complete, and concurrent treatment of both disorders. This tertiary level is generally a highly specialized unit and is not readily available in most communities.

This scarcity of tertiary centres has generated huge challenges for patients and treatment centres alike. Because individual clinicians have not been adequately trained, and medical systems have not been well-enough organized, concurrent disorders have not been addressed in an integrated fashion. Thus, patients suffering from concurrent disorders have been required to obtain treatment for each disorder from separate clinicians or systems. It has not been uncommon for a patient to obtain treatment at the local alcohol and drug treatment program and separate treatment for a mental illness through the mental health system. This has led at times to contradictory treatment approaches or recommendations, and the prescription of addictive medications to treat the psychiatric disorder.

Lower-level residential settings must now manage more complex psychiatric disorders, often in the absence of any specialized program and trained professionals, and in a milieu that is not designed for this level of psychiatric acuity. The result is a frustrating experience for patients, family members, and staff, and a disruption of the treatment program generally.

Over the last several years, the delivery of services has continued to improve. Increasingly, treatment is provided in an integrated "one-stop shopping" approach, rather than the previous sequential or parallel treatment process. Availability of integrated treatment varies considerably, however, and there is still significant room for improvement.

Clinical Challenges

Major Depression

Major depression is common in the population generally; approximately 10 percent of men and 20 percent of women will experience a major depressive episode during their lifetime, and most will experience recurrences after that. People suffering from major depression have an elevated risk of developing a substance use disorder. Explanations for this differ. There may be a shared genetic or developmental vulnerability leading to the development of both disorders. Another common explanation involves the self-medication hypothesis, which argues that people use alcohol or drugs as a means of coping with depression and its symptoms. For example, people may use marijuana or alcohol to "medicate" their insomnia, or cocaine or other stimulants to "medicate" their low energy. Getting drunk can be an escape from the experience of depression or sadness. An erroneous assumption often made by mental health professionals is that in treating "the cause" – in this case, the depression – the addiction issues will resolve without treatment. In fact, both disorders require treatment.

In spite of the elevated risk of substance use disorders in people who also suffer from depression, the reality is that most people with substance use disorders and comorbid depressive symptoms have a primary addiction problem. The depressive symptoms will improve significantly or remit when the addiction is arrested. This has been well documented in research with respect to alcoholism and comorbid depressive symptoms. For example, in one study, 42 percent of male alcoholics met the criteria for depression on admission. This was down to 6 percent by the end of the fourth week with abstinence alone. The largest reduction in depressive symptoms occurred by the second week (Brown and Schuckit 1988). A similar pattern has been observed for other substances, although this is less extensively researched. With stimulant drugs such as cocaine, crack cocaine, and methamphetamine , there may be a down regulation of the reward centre which may take several months to normalize, leading to a state of reduced pleasure generally. This is demonstrated in a recent review of anhedonia (the inability or reduced ability to experience pleasure) in people suffering from substance use disorders (Garfield et al. 2014). This review found that anhedonia was elevated across a range of substances, and typically appeared as a consequence of substance dependence. Patients on long-term opiates are also at significant risk of depression that often improves with abstinence.

After addicts have gone through the acute withdrawal syndrome, they may experience *postacute withdrawal,* an important concept in the field of addiction. This phase, where lower grade, longer-term withdrawal symptoms continue to persist, can last several months into abstinence from alcohol and various drugs. The symptoms often include various mood disturbances, insomnia, cognitive issues, and other problems with affect regulation.

Nunes and Levin (2008) from Yale University have researched co-occurring depression and addiction for several years. In one study, they focused on the treatment of depressive symptoms in patients who continued to actively drink and use drugs. Their findings suggested that patients might experience some relief from their depressive symptoms by taking antidepressants, even when they actively continued to drink alcohol. In those studies where antidepressants were noted to be helpful, patients were able to reduce their alcohol consumption, although complete abstinence was unlikely; this reflected a further need for specific addiction treatment.

In contrast, research does not generally suggest benefits from antidepressant treatment of depressive symptoms in the context of active stimulant and opiate dependence. While there may be individuals who do receive some benefit, the data did not suggest this across the board. Once again, even if depression is the identified concern, any clinical encounter provides an opportunity to work with motivation for treatment of addiction as a means to improve depression and mental health generally.

A common clinical challenge is in managing antidepressant treatment in the first several weeks of abstinence. In this early phase of abstinence, a significant proportion of alcoholics who appear depressed on admission will spontaneously improve. Initiating antidepressant treatment at this time might lead to exposing someone to medications that are not required. Generally, if possible, it is best to wait at least a couple of weeks before initiating treatment with antidepressants. Earlier treatment may be considered if there is a clear history of previous depression in the absence of addiction, if depressive symptoms are more severe, or if there is a significant family history of depression or mood disorders. It is not uncommon for patients to enter treatment having already been started on antidepressants by a family physician or psychiatrist. That treating clinician may not have enquired about the presence of addiction; alternatively, the patient may have minimized the situation or deliberately deceived the clinician. With a reasonable dose and passage of time, consideration could be given to stopping the antidepressant, particularly if the individual improves with abstinence. If there is an obvious benefit to antidepressants, in spite of a person's active drinking and drug use, it may be beneficial to remain on the antidepressant for the first year of recovery and abstinence, and then to reconsider the necessity of an antidepressant with an appropriate clinician.

In long-term abstinence, people continue to run a somewhat elevated risk of depression in spite of not using alcohol and drugs. Antidepressant medication can be prescribed as under normal conditions.

Some clinicians have tried matching specific antidepressants or classes with specific patients. Some recommend the use of more sedative-type antidepressants for people who are addicted to a more sedative class of drug, such as alcohol and opiates. Conversely, more stimulant-type medications are sometimes administered to those who are addicted to stimulant drugs such as cocaine or methamphetamine. Additionally, a subgroup of opiate addicts suffer from pain conditions, for whom SNRIs (such as Effexor or Cymbalta) are sometimes specifically recommended. SNRIs appear to have the benefit of reducing pain, in addition to treating depression. Alternatively, in early recovery, people may undergo particular struggles that may preferentially respond to specific types of antidepressants. For example, some patients with postacute withdrawal will describe difficulties with energy and cognition, so a more stimulant-type antidepressants may be helpful. Some patients with ADHD, who have abused psychostimulants, may benefit from a stimulant-type antidepressant if they have concurrent depression.

That said, the most potent antidepressant for most patients is active engagement in the recovery process, typically through a twelve-step program such as Alcoholics Anonymous or Narcotics Anonymous, with or without the process of residential treatment (see chapter 7, Twelve-Step Approaches, and chapter 10, The Course of Treatment). This process provides people with the necessary social connections and support to walk through the process of shame and guilt related to the disease of addiction. The outcome of addiction, of course, is that people hurt those who they love the most, and this can be very difficult to face after years of addiction to alcohol and drugs. However, I have observed a number of patients whose chronic depressive syndromes have improved substantially through residential treatment of addiction. This is often accomplished by addressing resentment, self-pity, and the sick role. At times, patients appear to be able to reframe their problems and have a more positive outlook. Regular exercise, proper sleep hygiene, and good nutrition practices are also very important.

As well as generating significant mood symptoms, grief and loss often trigger the addictive process. These are illustrated in the case of Rebecca, below.

Bipolar Disorder

Two facts warrant special attention at the beginning of this section. The first is that 50 to 60 percent of patients with well-documented bipolar disorder have a significantly elevated risk of having a substance use disorder, which in turn is associated with a worsened clinical outcome (Chengappa et al. 2008; Ostacher 2011). The second however, is that most patients with substance use disorders who experience mood swings do *not* have bipolar disorder!

Unfortunately, many patients with addiction are inappropriately diagnosed with bipolar disorder and put on various medications, which can have a significant negative impact. The clinician may not have properly investigated for the presence of a substance use disorder or, alternatively, the patient may not have disclosed the extent of their use of various substances.

We need to recall that alcoholics and drug addicts generally work very hard to keep the extent of their addiction hidden from others. Over time, family and friends may observe significant changes in their relative's personality and behaviour, many of which can resemble bipolar disorder. We are in the era of the Internet. These well-meaning family members, unaware of the extent of their relative's addiction, may read about bipolar disorder, and conclude that the mood swings they observe are caused by bipolar disorder rather than addiction. Consider the many symptoms of hypomania or mania — increased energy, racing thoughts, impulsivity, increased sex drive, and increased spending. It is very clear that addiction is a good impersonator of mood disorder.

I recall a man who was admitted to our residential treatment program a few years ago for treatment of his alcohol dependence. He openly admitted that he had been encouraged to see his family physician by his wife, as she was concerned about significant mood swings, and had read about bipolar disorder on the Internet. He was a very heavy drinker at the time, much of it done in secret. He did not disclose the extent of his drinking to his doctor, and the doctor did not ask about his use of alcohol and drugs. As a result, he was started on divalproex as well as one of the commonly used atypical antipsychotics. Over the next several months, his mood state underwent no significant change. He gained approximately fifty pounds, became a noninsulin-dependent diabetic, and had elevations in his cholesterol and triglycerides. Completion of a detailed history revealed no clear indication of any hypomanic or manic episodes, in spite of his so-called mood swings. At this point, he openly discussed his use of alcohol. During treatment, his medications were gradually tapered. His moods became stable with no indication of depression or hypomania or mania. He continued to receive treatment for alcohol dependence and had an uneventful course of treatment. He said he felt considerably better being off medications, and he gradually lost some weight during the time that he was with us.

Accurate assessment and diagnosis is critical. It can be particularly helpful to focus on periods of abstinence, if these have been present in the past. A positive family history can also be helpful. Obtaining past psychiatric records from psychiatric admissions or assessments can be invaluable.

Prospective mood charting following detoxification and entry into early recovery is also extremely helpful.

Bipolar disorders can also be masked by addiction, so identifying and treating such masked bipolar disorders is very important. I had the pleasure of bumping into a patient whom I had treated about seven years previously. She had done extremely well and had remained clean and sober, and was still actively involved with her recovery program. During her initial inpatient assessment, I felt that she might have a bipolar disorder and was able to elicit a history of at least one manic episode. She had not been previously diagnosed or treated for this disorder, as her addiction was always felt to be the primary problem. She was started on mood stabilizers and she did well during inpatient treatment. Her moods became stable and remained so until she became pregnant, when she ended up having a postpartum mood episode. She was abstinent from alcohol and drugs at the time, so the episode was clearly part of her bipolar disorder.

Serious consideration needs to be given to medications selected for patients with concurrent substance use disorder and bipolar disorder. One potential risk in particular is cross addiction to benzodiazepines, which are frequently used in the management of bipolar disorder for insomnia, anxiety, or hypomania/mania. Atypical antipsychotics may be used temporarily in place of benzodiazepines. Quetiapine is a commonly used example, as it has some sedative qualities. (This is "off label" use and informed consent is required.) If benzodiazepines must be used, a longer half-life benzodiazepine such as clonazepam will have a lower risk of addiction than a short-acting benzodiazepine such as lorazepam, although both should be avoided if at all possible.

One sees an interesting constellation of drugs of choice and self-medication in the area of bipolar disorder. For example, some bipolar patients attempt to initiate a desired elevated state through the use of stimulants such as cocaine, while others may drink alcohol to sleep when they are in a hypomanic or manic state. Others will use cocaine for energy and mood elevation when they are depressed, or drink to escape the pain of their depression. Generally speaking, alcohol and marijuana are the most frequently abused drugs in bipolar disorder; a subgroup of people abuse cocaine, crack cocaine, or various other drugs.

Psychosis

Psychotic symptoms are clearly a complication of alcohol and drug use, particularly with stimulant drugs such as cocaine, crack cocaine, and methamphetamine. More recently, a class of drugs commonly referred to as "bath salts" have been highlighted in the media. Very high-profile incidents have resulted from psychotic behaviour attributed to this class of drug. There has also been considerable interest in the association between marijuana use and transient or longer-term psychotic symptoms. The most significant classes of drugs and their association with psychotic symptoms are reviewed below.

Alcohol. Alcohol is most commonly associated with depression and anxiety, withdrawal syndromes, and alcohol withdrawal delirium. Another syndrome, alcoholic hallucinosis, is most often seen with abrupt reduction or cessation of use of alcohol. The syndrome is primarily characterized by paranoid delusions and auditory hallucinations. It is distinguished from DTs by the presence of a clear sensorium. There is no disorientation as to person place or time, in contrast to DTs. This can be a very striking syndrome and typically requires treatment with antipsychotic medications.

Marijuana. Many individuals experience paranoia while using marijuana. This is a common reason for not continuing to use marijuana following early experimentation. It is also a reason that people give for quitting marijuana after more regular use. Clinicians have commonly observed that patients with more serious and persistent mental illness (such as schizophrenia or more severe bipolar disorder) who smoke marijuana on a regular basis may experience an acute exacerbation of their ongoing psychotic symptoms.

One of the recent trends in management of psychotic disorders has been the identification and aggressive case management of first-onset psychosis. There is a very high prevalence of regular marijuana use in this population. Over the last decade, considerable research has been done to explore the relationship between early and heavy use of marijuana and the subsequent development of psychotic disorders, to determine whether marijuana in fact is a cause of schizophrenia or other chronic psychotic disorders. A newer synthetic form of cannabinoid, " Spice," may be even more likely to cause psychotic symptoms. Many studies have suggested that marijuana is a risk factor for developing psychosis; however, one recent study concluded that "having an increased familial morbid risk for schizophrenia may be the underlying basis for schizophrenia in cannabis users and not cannabis use by itself" (Proal et al. 2014). Pro-marijuana groups have been very excited by this research.

In contrast, a presentation at the recent American Psychiatric Association conference by Dr. Michael Compton reported preliminary data from the Allied Cohort on the Early Course of Schizophrenia II project. It showed that youth who used cannabis between the ages of fifteen and seventeen experienced their first psychotic episode almost four years earlier than counterparts who did not use cannabis (Anderson 2014). Marijuana dose was also identified as a risk factor.

Further research is clearly required!

In spite of this recent research, a strong clinical argument can obviously be made for working with patients to significantly reduce or abstain from using marijuana, particularly if they experience worsening of their psychotic symptoms.

Stimulants. Stimulant drugs such as cocaine, crack cocaine, and methamphetamine are strongly associated with psychotic symptoms (see chapter 3 for a full description of these drugs).

Cocaine is widely available in almost any community in North America. Some people are very vulnerable to experiencing psychotic symptoms with even minimal use of the drug. Conversely, some extremely heavy crack cocaine users report few psychotic symptoms. Typically, escalating risk of developing psychotic symptoms is associated with quantity and frequency of use, and the extent of sleep deprivation. It is not unusual for cocaine and crack cocaine users to binge-use, over a period of two or three days or longer. As the binge progresses, they describe increasing symptoms of paranoia, often feeling that they are being followed or watched. At times they may arm themselves with various forms of weapons for self-protection. Some cocaine and crack cocaine addicts report an almost contagious quality to the psychotic symptoms; they can become paranoid if they are around others who are experiencing paranoia. Typically, any psychotic symptoms improve dramatically when they stop using, or sleep. Much milder paranoia may continue for a few days, however. Some individuals will continue to experience prolonged psychotic states, with severe symptoms mimicking naturally occurring psychotic disorders.

Methamphetamine may generate psychotic symptoms more strongly, and the symptoms may last several days or weeks. There are a number of reports of very long-standing psychotic disorders resulting from methamphetamine use (Grelotti et al. 2010; Lecomte et al. 2013). In these prolonged psychotic states, it is difficult to determine whether what is happening is a methamphetamine-induced psychosis or whether the drug has triggered a psychotic reaction in someone who had the vulnerability. Research has shown that a family history of psychotic disorders is a predisposing risk factor for developing psychotic symptoms following methamphetamine dependence. Interestingly, nonspecific neurological factors also appear to be a risk factor, in the absence of a family history. This may include learning disabilities, ADHD, and prior head injury. Patients may well require psychiatric admission and treatment with antipsychotic medications.

One of the challenges for law enforcement has been the phenomenon of designer drugs, generated by slightly modifying known psychoactive drugs, which are not specifically illegal. The drugs are then marketed for uses such as "bath salts" or "deodorizers," with specific directions to not use internally, yet with a target audience that will clearly use them in this fashion. As noted, several high-profile incidents have been associated with the use of these "bath salts," drugs in the cathinones family (a type of amphetamine) that essentially function as stimulants. This class of drugs has led to severe psychotic reactions, with well-publicized harmful effects.

It is interesting to consider some of the underlying neurobiological processes associated with the use of stimulant drugs. Initial use of stimulants leads to dramatic escalations in dopamine in the reward areas of the brain. This is experienced subjectively as a powerful euphoria or high. As drug use is continued, the brain attempts to maintain its normal equilibrium by buffering these significant changes in dopamine activity. As a result there are both quantitative and qualitative changes in dopamine receptors which fight the action of the drug, leading to the development of tolerance or an increasing difficulty in obtaining the original high. Conversely, the opposite process occurs in two important areas. The first is in the area of craving or wanting the drug. This characteristic escalates over time, consistent with sensitization or kindling. In a similar fashion, once a stimulant addict begins to experience symptoms of psychosis, this pathway becomes increasingly entrenched and eventually replaces the previous euphoria or high. Addicts are then in the catastrophic position of wanting a drug badly enough to give up everything in their lives they value, in order to obtain a drug that no longer gives any significant or sustained elated mood state, but consistently leads to escalating psychotic symptoms and paranoia.

Anxiety

Management of anxiety symptoms and anxiety disorders is a very important theme in concurrent disorders. The relationship between substance use disorders and anxiety symptoms and disorders stand out in several important ways, as follows.

1. Anxiety disorders are often present prior to the development of substance use disorders. In efforts to self-medicate, people select substances they know will reduce their anxiety symptoms. In a very

common example, people who suffer from social anxiety have long known that alcohol is a very helpful social lubricant. If they have a vulnerability to addiction, concurrent disorders can result. A similar process is seen with patients suffering from posttraumatic stress disorder.

2. Anxiety symptoms are a common complication of withdrawal, particularly from alcohol, benzodiazepines, and opiates. If the symptoms cannot be appropriately managed, patients frequently leave treatment and return to their drug of choice.

3. Anxiety symptoms are also a feature of intoxication with certain drugs and can therefore mimic certain anxiety disorders, leading to inappropriate treatment by well-intentioned clinicians, who fail to treat the underlying addiction.

4. Anxiety symptoms or disorders may prevent patients from accessing treatment resources, particularly twelve-step treatment group therapy programs such as Alcoholics Anonymous or Narcotics Anonymous.

Approximately one-quarter of individuals with anxiety disorders suffer from comorbid substance use disorders. All the major anxiety disorders overlap in specific ways to substance use disorders.

Panic Disorder with or without Agoraphobia

A number of patients will experience apparent panic attacks while intoxicated with stimulants and this is also regularly reported by some patients using marijuana, in spite of its reputation as a sedative.

Alcohol withdrawal can mimic the symptoms and presentation of panic attacks. I once treated a middle-aged woman who worked during the day and drank heavily in the evenings. She had been diagnosed as having panic disorder in the recent past and was on antidepressants for this, however she reported no previous history of significant anxiety or panic attacks until the past year or so. She would generally feel well in the morning, but as the day progressed she became increasingly anxious, and described what she felt were panic attacks by afternoon. These panic attacks were immediately relieved when she would start drinking alcohol in the evening. It became clear to me that her symptoms were actually alcohol withdrawal, which was becoming increasingly problematic between drinking episodes. The panic attacks stopped with abstinence.

People who suffer from recurrent panic attacks and agoraphobia often describe the significant relief that drinking alcohol provides. Before leaving the home or going into various situations that would normally provoke anxiety, such as shopping, banking, driving, or crossing bridges, they will use alcohol to calm themselves down.

Addiction to alcohol is a risk factor for cross addiction to other substances such as the prescription benzodiazepines that are commonly used to treat anxiety disorders. Alcoholics treated for anxiety disorder may be put at risk of becoming addicted to the benzodiazepines used to treat the disorder, complicating the substance use disorder.

Benzodiazepines have been used for many years as a fast-acting, effective treatment for a variety of anxiety disorders. Most best practice guidelines suggest short-term use only, but some people remain on these medications for many years. Unfortunately, people who are vulnerable to addiction may begin to experience tolerance, needing escalating doses, and eventually becoming physiologically dependent. Benzodiazepines can be extremely difficult to withdraw from. Protracted withdrawal syndromes are common, so addicts need a very extended gradual withdrawal process, under ideal circumstances (see Ashton 2002).

Many residential treatment programs and detoxification units take a considerably more rapid approach than programs based in the community. At a very busy "cake night," my first at Edgewood, where patients celebrate various landmarks in recovery, I recall how the meeting was interrupted by a young woman having a seizure. She had had no history of seizures and had been uneventfully detoxified from alcohol the week before. However, she reluctantly disclosed that she had secretly been using significant amounts of benzodiazepines; her seizure was a symptom of benzodiazepine withdrawal. We were then able to detoxify her appropriately.

Original anxiety symptoms may recur or even be amplified through a rebound process, making withdrawal very uncomfortable. Other classes of nonaddictive medications may be used, off indication, with appropriate informed consent, for successful management of these symptoms. Examples are low-dose atypical antipsychotics or Gabapentin.

Social Anxiety Disorder

Social anxiety disorder, a common form of anxiety disorder, can be particularly problematic in substance use disorders. Most of us have experienced the relaxation and social disinhibition associated with using alcohol in social situations. Individuals with social anxiety disorder may be particularly aware of this benefit! It is not uncommon for them to drink before and during social encounters, in order to reduce their anxiety and enhance socialization. Once again, if there is a predisposition to addiction, this can lead to escalating alcohol consumption and a comorbid condition of social anxiety disorder with alcohol dependence.

Generally speaking, treatment of social anxiety disorder involves medications and/or cognitive behavioural approaches. Various antidepressant medications have been shown to be beneficial for treatment of social anxiety disorder. Benzodiazepines are commonly used as well, either situationally or on a regular ongoing basis, with the caveats described above.

Management of social anxiety can be very important in terms of outcome and prognosis. The treatment of addictions generally involves social activity. In the context of residential addiction treatment, social anxiety disorder may initially be extremely distressing, as one is required to engage in various group therapy modalities. Some may find it extremely difficult to engage in group therapy and therefore obtain its benefit. For the same reason, attendance at twelve-step meetings such as Alcoholics Anonymous or Narcotics Anonymous can be very problematic for someone with social anxiety. If social anxiety is not adequately treated and social activity is avoided, the self-medication process may continue and the risk of relapse may be escalated. On the other hand, if group therapy can be reasonably tolerated, it becomes a form of exposure therapy to group situations and ideally can lead to some habituation and lessening of the anxiety response with time. Another strategy is to connect the individual with social anxiety disorder with another member of Alcoholics Anonymous prior to attending meetings, for support.

Posttraumatic Stress Disorder

The identification and management of trauma and its sequelae is recognized as an important area in addiction treatment. Dr. Gabor Maté, a Canadian physician and author of *In the Realm of Hungry Ghosts*, has been a particularly strong advocate of this perspective. Prolonged exposure to trauma often precedes the development of addiction. As well, the addictive process and its associated lifestyle may also cause exposure to trauma. A number of individuals who are exposed to trauma will develop posttraumatic stress disorder (PTSD).

There are numerous best practice guidelines specifically for PTSD (Benedek et al. 2009; Bisson et al. 2005, 2007, 2013; Canadian Psychiatric Association 2006; Foa and Keane 2008; Forbes et al. 2007; Hamblen et al. 2009; Institute of Medicine 2008; National Collaborating Centre for Mental Health 2005). I reviewed a number of these in preparation for a series of lectures I gave on PTSD and addiction between 2007 and 2012 at various annual conferences on addiction medicine and PTSD.

In general, the results were remarkably consistent. In terms of medications, the results were generally favourable for SSRIs, SNRIs, some tricyclics, and augmentation with atypical antipsychotics. Prazosin was helpful for sleep problems in PTSD. Propanolol showed conflicting results and anticonvulsants generally had insufficient evidence. Benzodiazepines were shown to have a negative effect. A variety of psychotherapy approaches were also shown to be very effective, including prolonged exposure, trauma-focused cognitive therapy, and eye movement desensitization and reprocessing therapy (EMDR). There also appeared to be a nonspecific positive effect from various group therapies, with somewhat mixed results.

A much less clear picture is available when one is looking specifically at PTSD in conjunction with a comorbid substance use disorder. A few of the best practice guidelines make specific reference to this scenario. Both the British (National Collaborating Centre for Mental Health 2005) and Australian (Forbes et al. 2007) guidelines recommended treatment of addiction first, if comorbidity was present. However, one report sounds this cautionary note: "the literature is almost completely uninformative about how best to treat the substantial portion of veterans who have an important comorbid condition [in reference to PTSD and addiction]" (Institute of Medicine 2008). Two reports state that exposure therapy is risky, is not recommended, and may in fact have negative results (Health Canada 2002; SAMHSA 2008). Several guidelines mentioned Seeking Safety, the well-established structured treatment program for comorbid PTSD and substance abuse, as the only recommended treatment for PTSD and comorbid substance use disorders. This program was developed by Dr. Lisa Najavits from Harvard University (Najavits 2002). It has been widely used and definitely does not incorporate exposure-based treatments.

However, a number of experienced clinicians and researchers have been studying the effect of exposure-based therapies relatively early in recovery. One example is the Concurrent Treatment of PTSD and Substance Use Disorders using Prolonged Exposure (COPE), a structured thirteen-session treatment approach (Mills et al. 2012). Some positive results are being seen; these should generally be approached with caution. Exposure treatments should be introduced gradually, if they are going to be used. Importantly, before entering exposure-based treatment, people need to have established a support network, and they also need a reasonable skill set in terms of maintaining abstinence in recovery. If the trauma is more isolated and circumscribed, management is likely to be less complicated than long-standing historical exposure to trauma in various forms.

In summary, PTSD treatment best practice guidelines are very clear and well documented when this condition is present in isolation. When it is complicated by comorbid substance use disorders, the picture is much more cloudy. The best documented treatment is Najavits's Seeking Safety, a nonexposure-based treatment. Exposure treatments, which have the immediate effect of escalating anxiety and distress, may be risk factors for relapse into alcohol and drugs.

While many of the guidelines available are somewhat dated, they appear consistent with more recent suggestions. For example, a recent *Medscape* article suggests that "treatment is often complicated by comorbid disorders. If present, alcohol or substance abuse problems should be the initial focus of treatment" (Gore 2014).

Eating Disorders

Eating disorders include anorexia nervosa, bulimia, and binge-eating disorder. Canadian statistics suggest that the lifetime prevalence of anorexia nervosa is almost 1 percent in women and .3 percent in men. This increases in bulimia to 1.5 percent of women and .5 percent of men. The lifetime prevalence of binge-eating disorder is estimated to be 3.5 percent of women and 2 percent men (Hudson et al. 2007). Anorexia nervosa and bulimia nervosa are well-established psychiatric diagnoses; binge-eating disorder was added as a diagnosis in the DSM-5. Many studies have reported that eating disorders and substance use disorders frequently co-occur, although the specific rates vary considerably between studies. Some have suggested that these disorders may share a genetic link, accounting for part of the comorbidity ("Alcohol Abuse, Eating Disorders Share Genetic Link" 2013).

The extent to which eating disorders share common clinical features and underlying neurobiology with addiction disorders has been thoroughly discussed. Recently, for example, a thoughtful article on the addictive dimensionality of obesity, in which excessive consumption of food was linked with the reward circuitry of the brain, has been published by Dr. Nora Volkow and colleagues (Volkow, Frieden et al. 2013). Dr. Volkow is a well-recognized expert in the neurobiology of addiction. Caroline Davis (2013) has also considered the overlapping symptoms and characteristics of binge-eating disorder and models of food addiction.

Anorexia nervosa patients are driven by a pursuit of thinness and weight loss. They have major body image distortion, seeing themselves as overweight or overly large in spite of any objective evidence to the contrary. They are typically phobic of gaining weight and much of their mental life is preoccupied with weight, body image, and food. This leads to significant restriction of food intake, as well as a driven attempt to burn off calories through excessive exercise and use of medication such as stimulants, laxatives, or diuretics. Anorexia inevitably leads to significant deterioration in health and has been estimated to have a 10 percent ten-year mortality. In general, anorexics exhibit significant denial regarding the presence of a disorder and see their behaviour as a solution rather than a problem. They are often forced into treatment with little motivation to change their behaviour. Because they see alcohol as a source of calories, patients with anorexia nervosa may have lower rates of alcohol use disorder than the general population.

Bulimia nervosa is primarily characterized by binge eating, typically of very large quantities of high-calorie food, and purging behaviours such as self-induced vomiting or the use of diuretics and laxatives. This is typically followed by feelings of guilt and shame and may lead to periods of restricting food intake. Bulimics have a feeling of loss of control, reflected in their uncontrollable eating. Unlike patients with anorexia nervosa, this state is often psychologically distressing and there is more motivation to try and eliminate the behaviour, although they also tend to have body image distortion and are also phobic of gaining weight. Binge episodes may be associated with emotional distress or various internal and external triggers, and in that sense share common features with substance use disorders.

Binge-eating disorder is also characterized by frequent episodes of uncontrollable binge eating leading to distress, guilt, shame, and self-loathing. Unlike bulimia, however, there are no regular attempts to purge, restrict, or use excessive exercise.

Bulimia nervosa and binge-eating disorder features lend themselves to application of an addiction treatment model, even though they are not generally considered to be addictions per se. They are experienced as distressing and lead to perceived negative consequences, factors generating a motivation for change. The concept of triggers (including various emotional states such as sadness, guilt, anger, loneliness, and rejection, or external triggers such as specific adverse life events) as leading to the problem behaviour (substance use, bingeing, or purging) is relevant to all three of these conditions. As a result, various approaches that can be used to manage emotional dysregulation or stress can be beneficial in managing all these behaviours. Additionally, the concept of abstinence, which is used in twelve-step programs routinely, can also be applied to bulimia in particular and to a lesser extent with binge-eating disorder. The unique challenge for eating disorder patients is that they cannot abstain from food and they are therefore in a very difficult position of controlling their food intake. Karen's case history, below, illustrates many of these points.

ADHD

The prevalence of ADHD in patients with addiction is significantly higher than in the general population. A recent review estimated that ADHD is present in almost one out of every four patients with substance use disorders (VanEmmerik-vanOortmerssen et al. 2012). In many ways, this is not surprising as elevated impulsivity is a core feature of ADHD and an obvious risk factor for addiction. The authors noted that cocaine dependence was associated with lower ADHD prevalence than alcohol dependence, opioid dependence, and other addictions. The finding is somewhat surprising, since some clinicians feel that some patients using cocaine may be self-medicating their ADHD symptoms with the stimulant effects of cocaine. Generally speaking, children and adolescents with ADHD have a significantly elevated risk of developing problems with addiction to alcohol and drugs. They also tend to have more behaviour problems at school, and may not experience as much success in academic performance, which may cause a drift into a more drinking-and-drugging peer group for acceptance.

The relationship between ADHD/ADD and substance use disorders has recently been reviewed (Humphreys et al. 2013). The authors noted that ADD/ADHD was now diagnosed in 11 percent of schoolchildren, and the rates had increased 3 to 6 percent every year between 2000 and 2010. One of the major focuses of the review was to try and determine whether treating ADD/ADHD in childhood or adolescence with psychostimulants such as Ritalin or Dexedrine altered the risk of developing a substance use disorder. "The best evidence to date seems to suggest that treatment with stimulant medication has no substantial role in increasing or decreasing risk for the development of alcohol and drug problems" (Szalavitz 2013). There was some suggestion that treatment might reduce the risk for girls but not for boys.

This represents some change in thinking, as previous research suggested that treating ADHD would reduce the risk of developing addiction in the future. It is reassuring, however, to know that there is no elevated risk of developing substance use disorders as a result of childhood or adolescent exposure to psychostimulants.

Several scenarios involving ADHD/ADD and substance use disorder present themselves.

Scenario 1. A patient with a current substance use disorder describes a childhood history of diagnosis and treatment for ADD/ADHD, but is not currently taking medications for that. In this situation, it is important to attempt to clarify the means by which the original diagnosis of ADD/ADHD was made, and by whom—clinicians ranging from very qualified specialists to those with little experience may make such a diagnosis. Confirmation of the diagnosis is important. Diagnostic criteria can be reviewed with family members, and report cards and specialist reports, if available, can also be reviewed. Which medications were used, and whether there was a documented benefit, need to be clarified. Additionally, it is important to ascertain whether there was abuse or diversion of any medications that may have been prescribed.

With these things established, the next question is whether the current treatment is appropriate. Many patients are not interested in being on medication for ADHD, because they feel they have outgrown their ADHD or have significantly improved with age. Others will have an interest in pursuing medication treatment, particularly after some period of abstinence, to allow establishment of a baseline and therefore monitor improvement over time.

Appropriate selection of medication is an important consideration. Generally speaking, a nonaddictive medication such as atomoxetine (marketed as Strattera), indicated for ADHD, is a desirable first choice. Other nonaddictive options include various stimulant-type antidepressants which have been useful for some patients in the past. This is an off-indication use, as these medications are not specifically indicated for treatment of ADHD. Lastly, psychostimulant medications can be considered with careful review of risk-benefit issues. Ideally, selection of a long-acting formulation with associated reduced addiction risk is most appropriate. In this case, it is best to have well-established follow-up to document a positive response to medication as well as watching for any indication of relapse or diversion.

Scenario 2. There are clearly some patients whose addiction profile includes obvious abuse or diversion of psychostimulant medications. In my opinion, this is a clear contraindication to prescribing these medications and should be avoided. Atomoxetine and selected antidepressants with a research base could be considered.

Scenario 3. Continuing with the current treatment might be appropriate, if its effectiveness has been clearly demonstrated and if there is no prior history of abuse or diversion of the medication. Consideration could be given to changing to one of the nonaddictive treatment options. Again, this involves a risk-benefit discussion.

Scenario 4. Patients may present with a current substance use disorder and no prior history of assessment or treatment of ADD/ADHD. Family members, patients, or clinical staff may express concern about the possible presence of ADD/ADHD and request assessment. Well-established guidelines exist for assessment and diagnosis of ADD/ADHD, including the third edition of the Canadian ADHD practice guidelines have been published (Canadian ADHD Resource Alliance 2010).

It is important to note that adult ADD/ADHD is a continuation of childhood ADD/ADHD. It does not occur as a new disorder in adulthood. Therefore the initial focus should be on establishing the presence of a childhood disorder, before considering the current situation. Assessing current symptoms of ADHD will necessarily be more challenging in the context of active addiction or very early recovery. In general, nonaddictive options should be considered first and more long-acting psychostimulant preparations be considered afterwards.

Personality Disorders

I must confess I have always had difficulty in communicating about this disorder to patients. Imagine being told that your personality is "disordered"! Isn't this who we actually are—imagine being told that you are disordered as a person!

Psychiatry has talked about personality disorders for decades. The DSM-5 has continued with the previous ten types of personality disorder, with the same previous clusters, on the basis of some similarities between them. So what is meant by a personality disorder? As described in DSM-5, the key elements of a personality disorder are as follows:

1. A personality disorder is an enduring pattern of inner experience and behaviour. The pattern manifests in two or more of the following areas: thinking, feeling, interpersonal relationships, and impulse control.
2. This pattern deviates markedly from cultural norms and expectations.
3. This pattern is pervasive and inflexible.
4. It is stable over time.
5. It leads to distress or impairment.

There are four core features of personality disorders:

1. Rigid, extreme, and distorted thinking patterns (thoughts).
2. Problematic emotional response patterns (feelings).
3. Impulse control problems (behaviour).
4. Significant interpersonal problems (behaviour).

In the context of addiction, four of the personality disorders have a clearly elevated risk of being associated with substance use disorders and addictive behaviour. These are the so-called "Cluster B" personality disorders: narcissistic personality disorder, antisocial personality disorder, borderline personality disorder, and histrionic personality disorder. These disorders are clustered together on the basis that they tend to present with much more dramatic, emotionally labile, and erratic behaviours with major problems associated with impulse control and emotional regulation.

The *narcissistic personality disorder* is best characterized by one word: entitlement. People with this personality disorder tend to be quite grandiose in their assessment of various personal attributes and tend to feel special. "It's all about me" typically drives their behaviours, often with disregard of others. This attitude creates significant difficulties in their key relationships at home or in the workplace.

Much has been written about *antisocial personality disorder*. Dr. Robert Hare, a world-renowned Canadian researcher and writer in the area of antisocial personality disorder, developed the psychopathy checklist and has written several books on the subject (Hare 1991, 2003). While many antisocial personality disorder types end up in criminal and forensic settings, another subgroup finds itself in the upper echelon of businesses and corporations. Their pervasive pattern of disregard for the rights of others, at times manifesting with hostility or aggression, allows them to walk over others in pursuit of their own goals, with minimal empathy or guilt to interfere with their progress. Evidence of this personality disorder is often present in childhood, with histories of overt acts of violence, criminal activity, cruelty to animals, and fire settings; however the disorder can be much more subtle than this. Such people tend to be highly impulsive. They are often missing a moral compass and tend to blame others for things not working out in their lives.

People with *histrionic personality disorder* are very dramatic and visible. They tend to be highly attention seeking and emotionally overreactive; they are what we call drama queens. They are often described as shallow and lacking in substance.

There has been considerable interest in *borderline personality disorder* over the years and strong consideration has been given to the overlap with mood disorders. There has also been considerable debate in the psychiatric literature regarding the role of trauma in the development of this particular personality type. People with this disorder are well-known for their dramatic mood shifts, associated suicide attempts, and self-harm. They tend to exhibit impulsivity in a variety of areas, of which substance use is one. They have an unstable sense of identity and have a tendency to alternately idealize and then devalue others. Clinically, they are very good at generating double-binds, which place people (such as clinicians) in no-win situations. Probably the most popular treatment modality for borderline personality disorder at this time is DBT, originated by Dr. Marsha Linehan (Dimeff and Linehan 2008). Of particular relevance to this discussion is that DBT is often used in the treatment of addiction disorders as well.

There are several important issues to consider in the context of personality disorders and addiction.

First, people with personality disorders of the Cluster B type tend to have a higher incidence of addiction disorders. They experience elevated impulsivity, extreme mood fluctuations, and emotional responses, and their personalities tend to generate chaos and dysfunction, leading to significant stresses in their relationships at home and work. They often self-medicate in response to life stressors and intense emotional states. Substances may be used in the context of impulsive suicide gestures or attempts.

Secondly, many patients in the process of their addiction exhibit various emotional states and behaviours which mimic personality disorders. It is extremely important not to label someone with a personality disorder diagnosis without a very high level of confidence, as these labels can be difficult to shake and can be stigmatizing. Addicts who are addicted to street drugs may have no obvious history of personality issues until the beginning of their addiction, at which time they began to experience some deterioration in their personality and behaviour. Sometimes, patients appear very histrionic and attention seeking in the early recovery phase, again with no prior history; this behaviour may settle with further abstinence. Criminality and apparent antisocial behaviour may also become apparent as people progress in their addiction.

Thirdly, in my opinion and observation, a twelve-step program can be extremely beneficial for individuals with personality disorder or extreme personality traits in the Cluster B realm. Twelve-step programs have a very strong focus on personal responsibility and accountability in relationship management. The ability to honestly appraise the nature of one's relationship with others, and ultimately make amends for what one has done, becomes very corrective for many individuals with personality disorders. If they are able to connect with a sense of spirituality and morality, and become respectful and compassionate toward others, they have the opportunity to change the nature of their character and become much more functional.

Interestingly, twelve-step programs speak universally about character flaws and the responsibility to manage and change these. This becomes a normal part of being an addict in recovery as opposed to being labelled abnormal (personality disordered) by society or culture.

Fourthly, management of personality disorders can be very challenging in a private therapy or residential treatment settings. These behaviours can be very disruptive to others and adversely affect the therapeutic milieu in residential settings. People with these disorders may do poorly with the group therapy and rules that are characteristic of residential treatment settings.

Case Histories

In this section, you will be introduced to a number of patient stories that reflect the cross-section of addiction-related challenges that we encounter. These include both substance use disorders and behavioural addictions. While these are all patients who were admitted for residential treatment of addiction, other treatment options and considerations will be discussed as well. Various clinical details have been omitted or altered in order to protect the confidentiality of our patients.

REBECCA

Rebecca, fifty-six, had been with her second husband for fifteen years, following the death of her first husband after thirteen years together. She had three adult children. She had been working in her own business. She was not a drinker until her first husband tragically died, approximately seventeen years earlier. He had had an unexpected medical incident, and had been found in the garage by her son. A few months later her father passed away from cancer. Her ten-year-old brother had been killed in a motor vehicle accident years ago.

In this context of grief and loss, Rebecca began drinking heavily. She had never been a daily drinker, but now she drank every second or third day, gradually increasing the amounts of alcohol she consumed. She would drink to the point of intoxication and have a hangover the following day, such that she would not want to drink for the next day or two. This led to a repeated pattern of drinking every two or three days. Most recently, she had been consuming up to twenty-six ounces of hard liquor on those days, and routinely suffered blackouts. She had had an accumulation of negative consequences including injuries, social isolation, and arguments with her husband. A couple of years ago, she had been charged twice with impaired driving.

She had not previously had any treatment for addiction. There was no history of street drug use, addiction to prescription medications, or history of behavioural addictions.

Apart from issues related to grief, she had no other significant psychiatric history, no history of suicidal thoughts or attempts, and no eating disorders.

Rebecca stated that her maternal grandfather died of alcoholism. She was also concerned about her brother's drinking. Treatment was targeted toward both her addiction and depressive symptoms, with a particular focus on grief and loss issues.

KAREN

Karen, twenty-seven, worked as a server in a local nightclub. She had been with her current partner for the last seven months and had no children. She developed an eating disorder in her midteens, initially starting by restricting calories in order to lose weight, which she followed by developing the characteristic features of bulimia. She began having recurrent binges and self-induced vomiting, which she had talked about with her friends. She would occasionally exercise. She did not use laxatives or diuretics. She began drinking on weekends in high school and would typically drink to the point of significant intoxication, often with blackouts and vomiting.

At the age of nineteen she began drinking regularly, particularly when she began working as a server with regular access to alcohol. This led to drinking on an almost nightly basis, almost always to the point of intoxication. At some point, she was offered cocaine and appreciated the fact that it made her feel much more sober and in control, particularly when she had already been drinking excessively. She also observed that her appetite was considerably less. Her use of cocaine became more regular, to the point that she was using daily or almost daily, typically 1 to 2 g daily. Her boyfriend was not supportive of her use of cocaine and she made significant attempts to keep this activity hidden. She noticed that her weight began to drop as her appetite was regularly reduced.

Gradually, however, her use of cocaine progressively increased to the point that she was having functional impairments in her personal life and work, her finances were also significantly impacted, and she began to experience paranoia, which made her very uncomfortable. At this point in time, she presented to an addiction counsellor who subsequently recommended residential treatment for her cocaine and alcohol dependence.

Karen completed her early detoxification phase uneventfully. However, without using cocaine, her weight gradually began to increase, leading to significant distress. She became mentally preoccupied by body image and diet. This led to alternating attempts to restrict and subsequently binge and purge. This came to the attention of her counsellor and plans were initiated to implement a strategy for management of the concurrent disorder. This involved some initial discussion and education as to some of the shared features between her substance use disorder and eating disorder. These included the compulsive nature of the symptoms; the shame and guilt generated by these behaviours; the perceived value of secrecy and keeping the behaviour hidden; continuing the process in spite of negative consequences; and the need for abstaining from both alcohol and drugs as well as from purging behaviour, self-induced vomiting and using diuretics and laxatives.

A strategy was formulated to assist with the process. Karen would sit at the nursing station for a half hour after meals and use the time to journal about her feelings and emotions associated with eating and not purging. She explored triggers which typically led to use of drugs and also her eating disorder behaviour. With her counsellor, she discussed the application of the twelve-step process in terms of managing both conditions. Karen was assessed by both the family physician and psychiatrist. She used group therapy to gain insight into her emotions and feelings, establish trust, and make social connections — tools for obtaining support in the future.

JOHN

John, thirty, was single. He had no history of long-term relationships or children, which he attributed to extreme shyness and social anxiety. He had recently been terminated from his job in construction after ten months of employment. He had completed Grade 12. His parents remained together and he had three sisters.

John was admitted to residential treatment for treatment of alcohol, opiate, and benzodiazepine dependence. John stated that he began drinking at the age of eleven, stealing alcohol from his parents. By Grade 11 he was drinking six to eight beers on each of the three days of the weekend, typically alone at home and only rarely in social settings. He would typically go onto the Internet to listen to music or text. He reported he had drunk on a daily basis since the age of nineteen. His consumption had escalated; he was now drinking up to thirteen ounces of vodka daily, particularly when he was not working. His drinking was almost exclusively in isolation. He described blackouts. He had had one twenty-four-hour driver's licence suspension. He had lost jobs in the past as a result of his drinking and drug use. His family had been extremely concerned and he was estranged from his sisters. He had experienced significant withdrawal symptoms when he was not drinking.

John used other substances. He stated that he was a daily user of marijuana from the age of fifteen until finishing high school, at which time he stopped using it. He used dextromethorphan cough syrup occasionally during high school, and also used mushrooms.

At the age of eighteen, he was prescribed benzodiazepines for treatment of his social anxiety disorder. He recalls starting with a prescription for lorazepam 2 mg twice daily which he used excessively. He was switched to clonazepam while in a detoxification centre and was prescribed .5 mg tablets. Although he was prescribed four tablets daily, he was taking up to sixteen tablets daily. These were typically prescribed by a family doctor. He denied double doctoring, however he subsequently admitted that he was ordering benzodiazepines from the Internet as well as purchasing from street sources.

John stated that he met a friend while in detox who introduced him to heroin. He had begun smoking heroin on a daily basis for about two years. He had apparently quit, for approximately three months, and then picked up using once again, on a heavy daily basis, eight weeks before admission. He had injected heroin on a number of different occasions approximately six months previously. He had also abused a variety of prescription opiates at various times. He used cocaine once monthly at the age of twenty, however he generally did not appreciate stimulants. He denied any issues with gambling or sexually addictive behaviours. John was in a residential treatment program for three months in 2011. He relapsed almost immediately after completing treatment. In 2012, he was admitted to a psychiatric ward for two weeks, at which time he was tapered off benzodiazepines.

John stated that he had not previously had ongoing psychiatric care, apart from the detoxification on a psychiatric unit. He did have some counselling from a psychologist a couple of years previously. He said he had been taking Cymbalta 120 mg daily for the last five months, but later admitted that he had rarely taken it because of his ongoing drinking and drug abuse. He reported being on numerous antidepressants over the years, taking them inconsistently with no obvious benefit, which perhaps is not surprising.

He had read extensively on social anxiety disorder and clearly believed that he had this disorder. He also described being bullied a great deal over the years, which he attributed to his shyness and social vulnerability. This had become so bad in high school that he could only eat his lunch in the bathroom and was extremely stressed in school settings. He clearly described some unhappiness but generally did not see himself as depressed. There was no history of suicide attempts, although he had vague thoughts with no intent or plan of acting on these. There was no history of cutting.

He generally described a supportive family with no obvious trauma or abuse. He had an interest in jazz music and enjoyed time on his computer as well as watching TV and movies. He had always had a very limited social life as a result of his anxiety. His sisters were apparently much more outgoing and social.

John's grandmother was apparently addicted to prescription medications. He was not aware of any family history of mental illness or suicides. John described his father as a daily drinker for fifteen years until he developed gout three years previously, and quit drinking. The father said he felt much better after he quit drinking. His father allegedly did not receive any treatment for alcohol dependence and managed to abstain completely with significant improvements in his physical health, according to the patient. This is an example of someone who quit alcohol and drugs on his own, apparently successfully, without treatment.

John clearly described a pattern of alcohol and drug use consistent with dependence on alcohol, marijuana, benzodiazepines, and opiates. He appeared to have a family history of addiction. He also described a chronic problem with social anxiety disorder which appeared to predate his addiction. All of his drugs of choice were primarily downers, (having a significant sedative action), consistent with the concept that he started using these particular drugs of choice to self-medicate his anxiety disorder. I recall being very disturbed by his description of bullying in high school to the point that he would eat his lunch in the bathroom to avoid torment from other students. One can appreciate the perceived benefit of anything that would reduce these associated feelings of anxiety and distress that he was no doubt experiencing.

John also demonstrated a common phenomenon in addiction, cross addiction— addicted to one particular drug, he readily became addicted to another class of drug.

John obtained benzodiazepines from a variety of sources. Patients will sometimes obtain prescriptions from different doctors, to avoid detection of their excessive use. In this case, John obtained benzodiazepines from his family physician, but was also purchasing these medications from street sources as well as online pharmacy sources. British Columbia has a PharmaNet program allowing physicians to access information regarding filled prescriptions by patients. However, obviously PharmaNet would not have picked up his benzodiazepines from street and Internet sources.

I clearly recall talking to John about the treatment of his social anxiety disorder. He informed me that he had been taking Cymbalta 120 mg daily for the last five months. When I asked him if he was taking it regularly he stated "Yes—except when I'm drinking." When I pointed out that he was drinking every day he admitted that he had not been taking Cymbalta on any kind of regular basis. This illustrates one of the challenges of treating concurrent disorders.

John presented to treatment with physiologic dependence on three classes of drugs—alcohol, benzodiazepines, and opiates. He progressed in using all three drug classes to the point where he developed tolerance and ultimately dependence, causing significant withdrawal in the absence of the drugs. His initial detoxification had to take into account these three classes of drugs. The priority would be to address alcohol and benzodiazepine withdrawal, as these were the most dangerous, whereas opiate withdrawal would be uncomfortable but not dangerous. Since he was a young adult and had no known liver disease, and was withdrawing from benzodiazepines, a long-acting benzodiazepine was selected, in this case diazepam. He was placed on an extended benzodiazepine detoxification protocol, gradually tapering over four weeks.

Opiate withdrawal became an issue within twenty-four hours and Suboxone treatment was initiated for his withdrawal, according to our protocol. His maximal dose was 10 mg which was tapered over the following ten days. He was also provided with Maxeran to symptomatically treat gastrointestinal withdrawal symptoms, ibuprofen for muscle and joint discomfort, and Gabapentin to address anxiety related to withdrawal as well as his previous anxiety disorder, and insomnia.

TIM

Tim, twenty-nine, a university student, lived with his girlfriend in a major urban centre. He did not have children. Tim was admitted for residential treatment of methocarbamol dependence with a prior history of opiate, benzodiazepine, alcohol, and cocaine dependence, in addition to anabolic steroid use.

Tim began using opiates in Grade 10, starting off with Dilaudid and then using Percocet. He later progressed to OxyContin, which he was crushing and snorting, in doses up to 800 mg daily. He also began using alprazolam in Grade 12 and switched to diazepam, up to 150 mg daily. He began using cocaine at the age of eighteen and estimated using it monthly until the age of twenty-one.

He had been admitted to a residential treatment program three years ago, at which time he had been intranasally using 2 or 3 g of cocaine daily. He began drinking alcohol in Grade 8 and between the ages of nineteen and twenty-one was drinking three or four times weekly, at which time he would consume between thirteen and twenty-six ounces of vodka in addition to several beers. He was using marijuana but quit in Grade 12 as it made his anxiety worse. He was also using Ecstasy regularly in Grade 12, and had experimented with other drugs. He was admitted for residential treatment for four months in early 2011, approximately three years ago. He remained clean and sober, attending twelve-step meetings and working a successful recovery program. Approximately one year ago, he began taking Robaxacet for back pain and recalled that he had used this in the past for "a buzz" and began taking it in progressively larger amounts, to the point of taking fifty tablets daily. At the age of seventeen, and fairly regularly again in the previous year, he had also used anabolic steroids. He began smoking cigarettes at the age of twelve and had smoked regularly until the age of twenty-three .

He felt that he had a sex addiction. He described close to 100 partners. He routinely used pornography and prostitutes, and had a history of cheating on his girlfriends. He had been treated with a variety of psychostimulants for ADHD but generally did not like the feeling associated with these medications and denied abusing them.

Tim described a number of negative consequences from his use including blackouts and memory problems. He had experienced opiate withdrawal symptoms on several occasions as well as benzodiazepine withdrawal symptoms when these medications were not available. He had experienced paranoia when using cocaine. He had had a couple of serious legal charges. His school and social functioning had deteriorated significantly. He had been involved in selling drugs. He had lost a number of his friends and become estranged from family.

Tim reported having difficulties with depressive symptoms since childhood. These clearly worsened as his addiction progressed, prior to going into his first residential treatment. His mental status improved dramatically with abstinence and engagement in recovery, but his mood began to deteriorate once again, following his relapse. He had made two previous impulsive suicide attempts, while intoxicated. He had had thoughts about using carbon monoxide poisoning in the past. He currently stated he would not do this to his girlfriend or family. He was placed on an antidepressant prior to his first treatment but felt this was unnecessary after he had become clean and sober. He described himself as a perfectionist and felt he had some social anxiety, although this was generally mild. He also experienced some mild compulsive hand washing.

Tim had witnessed two separate friends being murdered. He also admitted to being sexually abused when he was much younger. He was apparently diagnosed with ADD by a psychiatrist at the age of six and again at the age of thirteen in another assessment. There was no history of psychiatric admission to hospital.

Tim stated that his paternal uncle was an alcoholic and addict. His paternal grandmother used opiates. His mother had a history of excessive drinking. His paternal uncle was a compulsive gambler and his paternal grandfather was an alcoholic.

Methocarbamol is a central muscle relaxant used to treat skeletal muscle spasms. It is better known as Robaxin. It has a mechanism of action which is very similar to benzodiazepines, barbiturates, the "Z" drugs such as zopiclone (Imovane) and zolpidem (Ambien), and alcohol. There are clearly reports of individuals becoming addicted to this medication, although it is not a common drug of abuse. This case again illustrates the concept of cross addiction, and reinforces the importance of avoiding medications or drugs which are known to cause addiction, even if the individual has not been addicted to that particular drug or class of drugs in the past.

Tim also exemplified a disturbingly common trend, the abuse of prescription opiates beginning during school years. These are often easy to access, since parents and relatives frequently have opiates in the home. Students are able to obtain these and share or sell them to friends. This has led to a dramatic escalation in the frequency of prescription opiate addiction, with development of tolerance and dependence. Once addicted, this becomes a very expensive habit. Rather than taking the pills by swallowing, they are frequently crushed and snorted to heighten the effect and facilitate a faster onset of action. They may also be dissolved and injected. One pattern that we are seeing clinically is initiation of prescription drug use until they can no longer be afforded or are not available, at which time the switch is made to heroin use. Heroin is widely available in most communities and is typically cheaper than prescription opiates.

Tim's history is fairly typical for an early onset, aggressive addictive disorder. He became addicted to a variety of drugs and drug classes, in addition to sexually addictive behaviours. Significantly, he was allegedly able to abstain from all addictive drugs, including opiates, for a period of two years while he participated in twelve-step programs. His relapse appears to have been triggered through the use of what would be considered a less addictive drug than prescription opiates, to manage a pain issue. It is interesting that his family history is characterized by a wide range of addictions. Also, in spite of his high propensity for addictive behaviours, associated with addiction to a variety of drugs and classes, he had no interest in abusing his psychostimulants. This is quite variable, as other addicts have clearly abused or diverted psychostimulants.

The concurrent disorder issue is interesting in Tim's case. While he described a history possibly consistent with dysthymia or mood disorder, we can see that he was abusing drugs from a very early age. One might have hypothesized that his mood disorder had led him to attempt self-medicate. If the focus had exclusively been on his mood disorder, the addiction would have been left untreated. In this case, abstinence, in addition to working a twelve-step recovery program, led to a dramatic improvement in the symptoms which were sustained until his later relapse.

The association of trauma and addiction is also clearly evident in Tim's story. He described being sexually abused at some point during his childhood and also witnessed two close friends' death. This is an extremely common finding in addiction treatment.

Individuals who have been very actively involved with the drug scene at the street level have typically been exposed to various forms of violence, at times leading to death, as well as accidental overdoses particularly from opiates and cocaine/crack cocaine. One innovative approach which is being explored, is the provision of a drug called naloxone to opiate-dependent addicts, which they can administer to other drug users if there is an accidental overdose and they stop breathing. This is another example of harm reduction, with the goal of saving lives during the course of active addiction.

LAURA

Laura, thirty-three, was a health care worker. She had been married for over a decade, and had three young children. She had been working full time, which involved some shift work. Laura was admitted to residential treatment for management of opiate dependence.

She first began using caffeine tablets in her early twenties, as a student, for energy. She had a history of occasional migraine headache and had been given a prescription for Tylenol 3 for this. She was immediately aware of a euphoric feeling, which she associated with her use of opiates. After her first child, she was given a prescription for Tylenol 3 when she returned home from the hospital. At that time she was also using caffeine tablets for energy. She admits to manipulating various doctors and friends in order to maintain a supply of opiates. She did not use street sources. She continued her opiate addiction by purchasing Tylenol 1, which did not require a prescription and could be obtained over the counter. She estimates taking twenty-five a day. She began to experience withdrawal symptoms when she tried to taper her quantities. She was seeing a neurologist but was not honest about her use of medication. She had also been using Gravol on a nightly basis for the last ten years, to help her sleep. She did not use street drugs. Laura had been a heavy weekend drinker in her teenage years, always drinking to the point of intoxication with hangovers, vomiting, and frequent blackouts. She quit for one year when she was dating a nondrinking, athletic boyfriend but returned to drinking when the relationship ended.

Laura described a turbulent adolescence, which she attributed to parental separation and conflict at home. She had been on Paxil, for five years which helped her anxiety. More recently she was taking mirtazapine with good effect. There was no history of suicidal thoughts or eating disorders. Laura was aware of a family history of domestic violence and addiction but no mental illness.

Chapter 10

Residential Treatment

A number of patients will be better suited to residential treatment than to outpatient or community programs, which they may have tried unsuccessfully in the past. This is particularly likely if they present significant withdrawal issues requiring medication and medical monitoring. Common examples would include people with alcohol dependence, benzodiazepine dependence, or opiate dependence, particularly if complicated by other medical or health issues. Other people may require residential treatment on the basis of the severity of their disorder, the absence of housing or social supports, complicating psychiatric disorders or symptoms, or the inability to attain sobriety for long enough to participate in community programs. Limited alternatives for community treatment in many geographic areas may also be a factor.

Residential treatment programs can be government funded or private. They range from very basic to very high end, with associated variations in cost. Ideally, a residential treatment program should have access to medical services. Some programs require withdrawal prior to admission, a two-step approach in which patients may get lost in the shuffle. There may be separate waiting lists for each component, particularly in government-funded programs. Psychiatric assessment and consultation are also extremely important, since addiction disorders are very often accompanied by mental health symptoms and disorders.

Residential treatment options vary considerably, although most are based on twelve-step facilitation therapy, which relies heavily on the twelve-step programs of Alcoholics Anonymous (AA), Narcotics Anonymous (NA), and various other programs for behavioural addictions. (See chapter 7, Twelve-Step Approaches, for a discussion of AA.)

The vast majority of residential treatment centres are abstinence-based. Their philosophy is to avoid all addictive medications and street drugs. This stance may cause distress for patients who are currently appropriately using potentially addictive medications for various illnesses, and are required to discontinue these. This is required to reduce the risk of developing cross addiction, wherein people cease using one addictive drug but transfer their addiction to another addictive substance. In these situations, nonaddictive medication alternatives are considered, to stabilize the medical condition or symptom. This is typically necessary for patients who are using benzodiazepines for insomnia or anxiety, or prescription opiates for pain. Patients are often confused and upset if they are asked to get off medications that they have been using—and not abusing—as prescribed. Education regarding the risk of cross addiction is very helpful in this regard..

The Tools of Residential Treatment

In twelve-step facilitation therapy in a residential setting, patients break out of the isolation of addiction and begin to connect socially with others. This most important and foundational aspect of the work allows people to see themselves as others see them. They learn to give and receive support. They begin to establish trust in others, and enhance their capacity for honesty and intimacy. They share a common struggle, and thereby become stronger; they experience "the power of We."

Medical Assessment

Ideally, a treatment centre will have access to medical assessment and treatment by a physician. Frequently, patients with severe addiction disorders will have neglected their personal care and avoided doctors, either out of neglect or embarrassment. As a result, some previously undetected medical problems, such as hypertension or diabetes, might surface. In addition, specific disorders caused by addiction, including various infectious diseases or liver disease, might be found. All need to be identified and treated.

Psychiatric Assessment

Patients with addiction disorders have a higher prevalence of psychiatric symptoms and disorders. Suicidality and violence toward others, increased with alcohol and drug addiction, also require psychiatric evaluation. Appropriate identification and treatment of concurrent disorders can lead to improved quality of life and reduced risk of relapse. Psychiatric assessment and treatment are therefore an important component of comprehensive care for individuals with substance use disorders. However, a limiting factor is that many treatment centres do not have direct, convenient access to psychiatric care.

Chaplaincy

While some patients in residential treatment programs have a well-established current or historical faith experience, many others struggle with the concept of spirituality and "God as you understand him." Well-informed and experienced chaplains have helped addicts of both kinds in their recovery.

Group Therapy

Group therapy teaches many skills: identifying feelings, establishing trust, sharing with others, and providing support. Because of the isolation and disconnection that are addiction's constant partners, this form of therapy is considered essential in the treatment of addiction. In group therapy, people begin to work through their shame and guilt through sharing experiences and feelings with others. Group therapy also provides the opportunity for group members to confront their disordered thinking and attitudes — "stinking thinking," as it's called in twelve-step programs — that are an obstacle to recovery. Many addicts find that they have repressed their emotions; these can be reclaimed through the group process.

Individual Therapy

There are often very sensitive issues associated with addiction, issues that may be extremely difficult to talk about in a group situation. Common examples might include a history of sexual abuse or sexual assault, spousal abuse, violence toward others, or graphically traumatic events that could potentially traumatize others, activating or reactivating their symptoms of PTSD. Some patients may require individual therapy if they are extremely shy or suffer from social anxiety disorder, although group therapy can act as a form of exposure therapy as well, treating the social anxiety disorder as a byproduct.

Lectures

Most residential treatment programs provide a series of lectures to increase understanding related to addiction and various aspects of recovery. These are generally provided by staff, but guest speakers may also be people in recovery who are able to share their own experience and hope.

Exercise and Diet

Most programs recognize the benefit of exercise as a step toward returning to improved physical health. Opportunities vary widely depending on the particular treatment centre and can be quite extensive in the more high-end private treatment programs. Consultation with a dietitian can also be very helpful, as nutritional health has frequently been poor prior to admission.

Assignments

Typically, numerous assignments can be used to help patients gain more insight into their own problems and increase their understanding of the disease of addiction. In the early stages, many assignments are focused on breaking denial and furthering an acceptance of the disease of addiction.

The Course of Treatment

In residential treatment programs, the treatment milieu itself-remains a powerful tool for recovery from addiction. Organizing and managing this tool is extremely complex and requires ongoing evaluation and review. Reinforcing the program's philosophy are many specific underpinnings, which may seem confusing and unnecessary to those who are new to the process. Many rules and expectations are involved.

Before Treatment

Patients typically become increasingly isolated as their addiction progresses. Their primary love relationship, in spite of their best intentions, is with their addictive substance. They repeatedly break numerous rules, both their own and others'. They draw a line in the sand, which they swear they will not cross, and then they cross it: reward = 1, judgment = 0. The winner becomes increasingly clear! Judgments generated in their brains have not taken them in a direction they would have wanted for themselves. Their physical health is often significantly impaired. Cognitive dysfunction is common during prolonged intoxication and withdrawal, and significant brain damage may also be caused by chronic substance use or other processes. As their addiction progresses, patients become increasingly detached from their own emotional states and find numerous ways to justify, rationalize, and deny the things going on in their lives.

During Treatment

At times, in treatment, patients see their situation with acute clarity, only to make a 180° turn the next day. "Judgment brain" becomes replaced by "reward brain," which then makes the decisions and choices. This process will continue for patients during treatment, so considerable efforts are made in treatment to engage judgment brain and suppress reward brain. Typically, this involves intense conversation with counselling staff, focused on activating judgment brain. Other patients with whom they have established a good relationship may be called in to assist as well. If this doesn't work, family and referral sources may be engaged through a crisis conference on the phone or in person, all with the intent of helping patients see the reality of their situation.

Responsibility and accountability have been missing at times in patients' lives prior to admission. Patients are therefore assigned various responsibilities in treatment, such as assisting in the kitchen and light housekeeping.

Throughout their treatment, efforts are made to provide patients with an interpersonal skill set that will allow them to handle the challenges they will face in recovery. Engagement with others and involvement in a supportive community are critical for helping develop these skills, which are often missing prior to treatment.

Inevitably, cravings appear and major stressors arise. These can trigger a relapse unless successfully managed. This means that patients actually need to be able to identify their own emotions, cravings, and need for help AND be able to communicate these effectively to others —a difficulty for many people suffering from addiction disorders. Foundational to this set of skills is building trust in others to provide accurate, helpful support. But trust is extremely difficult for many, depending on their childhood and subsequent life experiences. It involves considerable risk taking, and learning through experience that there are trustworthy people who can provide support. For this reason, the daily "feelings group" is a critical part of treatment.

No one entering treatment feels good about where their life has taken them. Bombarded by shame, guilt, and low self-esteem, people now find it difficult to see the good in themselves. Self-loathing may be particularly strong in early recovery. Treatment provides an excellent opportunity to receive feedback from others and learn about oneself, in spite of how difficult this process can be. A strength of group therapy is not only seeing the same addictive behaviours in other people, but also seeing the good in them — which may turn out to be a back-door route toward self-acceptance. Group also offers many opportunities to help and support others, which can be a powerful force in countering the trail of destruction of others that may have happened prior to treatment.

When patients enter treatment, they begin to give up addictive behaviours that have become their norm. As they seek to redefine "normal," many patients may experience a sense of reward deprivation, which they try to fill through other behaviours. Common examples include sexual flirting and acting out, spending, drinking excessive caffeine, bingeing on food, generating chaos, and expressing anger. These addictive equivalents are addressed in treatment, with the goal of finding constructive behaviours to replace them. Eating disorders may also become reactivated, particularly in women who have been addicted to stimulants on top of a prior history of eating disorder. Many patients may have used various solitary approaches to managing their emotions, such as playing guitar, listening to music, aggressive exercising, and journal or poetry writing. These otherwise healthy behaviours may be discouraged in the short term, to encourage patients to engage and to connect with others, instead of these more isolated approaches.

Spirituality is a strong component of twelve-step programs. This is often an early stumbling block for patients, who associate spirituality with religion, either from their past experience or their assumptions about what this will mean in treatment. A common way we deal with this concern in our treatment at Edgewood is by telling people: "It doesn't matter what your higher power is, as long as you recognize it's not yourself, and remember — your own best thinking got you here."

The first several weeks of treatment are primarily focused on breaking down denial, gaining insight, and recognizing powerlessness over addiction. When I first started working in addiction medicine, I remembered being shocked by how many alcoholics felt that they would be able to return to normal social drinking in the future. Not coming from an alcoholic family or having struggled with addiction myself, I felt that no one would ever want to return to anything that had caused so much harm and destruction. I also learned that many patients were interested in getting as close to the cliff as they could without falling off, rather than choosing a safer course of action. I was frequently reminded of this during my early days in addiction medicine. At that time, patients could go home on weekend passes. I was amazed at the number of patients who would come back on Monday proudly declaring that they had spent hours in the bar drinking only soft drinks, rather than avoiding this high-risk situation entirely.

Ideally, as the course of residential treatment progresses, several key problem areas are resolved. Detoxification is complete, physical health has been evaluated, and acute issues are stabilized. Follow-up may be organized for longer-term health issues. Patients will have had the opportunity to develop some of the communication skills required to transition to outpatient treatment such as twelve-step programs in the community. Families may have had the opportunity to do some of their own work, either independently or in association with the treatment program. People will generally have found their physical and mental health has improved significantly during this time. They may now be ready to return to many, if not all, major life functions at home and at work.

After Treatment

Patients will generally have been given an aftercare plan to follow after they return home. Following an aftercare plan is an essential part of good recovery. It typically involves various commitments:

- Attend three or more twelve-step meetings a week.
- Find a home group and sponsor (that is, a mentor in stable recovery).
- Attend individual counselling or aftercare meetings associated with the treatment program.
- Commit to abstinence and to maintaining a program for healthy sleep and nutrition.

Additionally, employees working in safety-sensitive positions or various specific professions may be required to engage in a mandatory random alcohol and drug screening program. A number of professions also provide self-help groups. These include the Caduceus group for health care professionals; Birds of a Feather for aviation professionals; and the Legal Profession Assistance Conference (LPAC) of the Canadian Bar Association, for lawyers.

Treatment Outcomes

What Works?

One of the most frequent and critical questions asked about any treatment of substance use disorders is "what is the success of your treatment?" This sounds as though it should be a simple question to answer. However, as it turns out, it is far more complex than meets the eye. William White (2012) has completed an exhaustive and excellent review of the issues.

One such issue relates to the definition of *success*, particularly as the term has been used in various research papers. Definitions of it vary widely; success has been studied using different criteria. In different studies, it may refer to complete abstinence alone, to no longer meeting clinical criteria for disorder, or functional improvement. These measures are ideally produced through self-reports, in addition to collateral information from other sources, including drug and alcohol testing, although these additional measures are frequently not used.

Studies show that different patient populations have different outcomes. Patients with less severe disorders who attend programs in the community are known to have different outcomes compared to patients with more complex problems who require residential treatment.

White estimates that anywhere from 5.3 to 15.3 percent of the general population of the United States is currently in remission from substance use disorders. Additionally, approximately 50 percent of individuals who met lifetime criteria for substance use disorders before treatment no longer meet those criteria. Interestingly, only 18 percent did so through a strategy of complete abstinence: "In the fifty adult clinical studies reporting both remission and abstinence rates, the average remission rate was 52.1 percent and the average abstinence rate was 30.3 percent" (White 2012, 2).

Similar findings were noted in the adolescent population. Another finding was that "of those who resume alcohol and other drug use following treatment, most do so in the first days and weeks. This finding underscores the need for and value of assertive approaches to posttreatment monitoring, support and early intervention for both adults and adolescents"(White 2012, 4).

Relapse

Addiction leaves a trail of destruction. The process of recovery, punctuated by frequent relapses, can be very challenging. It does not go in a straight line. I have repeatedly witnessed patients return for treatment who did well with their aftercare plan for a time, became overconfident, began to let their program go, and eventually relapsed. Once patients start consuming alcohol and drugs again, the addiction carries on where it left off; a new cycle of addiction begins.

Dealing with relapse can be very disappointing and a cause of much despair to addicts, their friends, and family. Experiencing a relapse to addiction following a period of sobriety, whether self-initiated or following intensive treatment, is typically very discouraging and demoralizing. The person who relapses experiences significant feelings of shame, guilt, helplessness, and hopelessness. Family members, friends, and employers are deeply affected, and once again everyone risks a further accumulation of negative consequences.

Relapse is a gradual process. Typically characterized by changes in motivation, attitude, emotions, thinking, and behaviours, it starts well in advance of when any addict begins to consume alcohol or drugs again. These are warning signs that relapse is occurring. Experienced clinicians and members of the recovery community are often able to identify these warning signs in advance, to help prevent actual use of alcohol and drugs.

Relationship issues may be a factor in relapse, either due to struggles with communication and intimacy, or being with a partner who uses alcohol and drugs or has relapsed in their own recovery. Other addictive behaviours such as gambling, sexually addictive behaviours, compulsive spending, or workaholism may also be observed prior to relapse to alcohol and drugs directly.

It is very important for addicts to understand their triggers, so that they can step back from the brink of relapse. There are three well-known triggers.

The first of these is *stress*. Instead of being overwhelmed by stress, addicts can learn how to metabolize it through individual practices such as relaxation, meditation, good nutrition, established sleep patterns, exercise, and maintaining strong social connections. Individual or group counselling, where various emotional triggers (such as resentment, anger, and frustration) can be identified and worked through, is a powerful means of stress management. This is a particular strength of twelve-step programs.

Meetings provide the opportunity to connect with others in a supportive, abstinence-oriented environment. Importantly, these programs encourage relationship with a sponsor, a person who functions as a senior mentor and who has struggled with similar issues earlier in their recovery.

The second major mechanism of relapse is *priming*, which may be thought of as priming the pump. Priming means exposure to any addictive drug that activates the reward centre from its more dormant setting. In this major mechanism of relapse, alcoholics begin to feel that they can return to moderate drinking— they can have "just have one drink." This is what AA might call "stinking thinking." This cognitive self-deception often leads to attempts to return to controlled use, and subsequently to out-of-control relapse.

Relapse may be to the original substance, such as alcohol, cocaine, or opiates, or exposure to a drug class not previously used. This often happens in a treatment setting, where benzodiazepines or opiates may be prescribed for insomnia, anxiety, or mood disorders. It is important to understand that *any* exposure to *any* addictive substance threatens the stability of an addict in recovery. If these medications are required for medical purposes, it is very important to enhance recovery activities and behaviours, and communicate this risk to the members of the person's support group.

The third major mechanism involves classic cues and triggers which have historically been associated with the person's use of alcohol or drugs. AA refers to this as *slippery people and places*. It is very important, particularly in early recovery, to avoid high-risk people and places. This is often a difficult lesson for people in early recovery. I recall, years ago, working in a facility where people were able to go home for the weekend during treatment. These individuals would describe, with great pride, how they spent the weekend at the bar but drank only soft drinks. It is amazing to me, even after years of working in the field, how patients can prefer to walk as close to the cliff edge as possible, rather than staying well back in safe territory, given the major losses they have experienced.

Restabilization is a critical component. The person may require withdrawal management once again. Housing and finances may be unstable. There may be new legal challenges. Clinical need and setting may need to be reassessed. An assessment of suicide risk is also very important, as patients are often very demoralized and hopeless at these times, particularly while under the influence of alcohol or drugs. One should be vigilant for any indication of untreated psychiatric disorders that may have been present during sobriety. Appropriate treatment of these disorders is obviously indicated.

Although relapse most frequently occurs within the first year of sobriety, it can happen at any point in one's recovery career. As noted, this is a devastating experience, particularly if one has years of sobriety and has garnered respect in the recovery community. This can be particularly difficult in the twelve-step community, where one may experience even more significant guilt and shame. Imagine someone who may have received their ten-year medallion, going up to get their first-day medallion weeks or months later. In these situations, it is very important to rigorously analyze the precursors to relapse. This provides a learning opportunity that may lead to an enhanced experience of recovery after the relapse, once other issues have been identified.

People in relapse may become entrenched in self-pity. It is very important to mobilize supports and resources, both internal and external. It is very important to remind them of the great successes they achieved leading up to their relapse, and consider how much more painful it would have been if they had been actively addicted instead, becoming progressively more unwell. I have repeatedly observed how a relapse can lead to a much more dedicated commitment to sobriety and recovery, and a subsequently enhanced experience of life.

Case Studies

HELEN

Helen, forty-five years old, was currently single. Five years ago, her ten-year marriage ended. She had no children. She had been employed for the last eighteen years.

Before treatment. Helen had used heroin and methadone for over three decades. Recently confronted by her employer, who also assisted her in getting into treatment, she was admitted for residential treatment of this opiate dependence. She first began using heroin at the age of sixteen, and stated that she was addicted by the age of eighteen. She had been an intravenous heroin user ever since, with no periods of abstinence, although she had made repeated attempts to reduce her use of opiates. In late adolescence she was introduced to methadone and had used methadone continuously while simultaneously using heroin. Typically, she said, she would take 50 to 70 mg of methadone daily. Most recently, she had been using a friend's methadone prescription. She had no significant history of prescription opiate use, and had never smoked opiates. In spite of three decades of addiction, she had not had any form of treatment other than the methadone.

She had not used cocaine or crack cocaine. She had done some drinking as a teenager but had used alcohol only minimally as an adult. She had at times been a regular user of marijuana. She stated that she had had the same heroin dealer for years and generally had not interacted with other opiate addicts for at least a decade. She denied problems with gambling or sexually addictive behaviours, and had no previous criminal charges. She was extremely anxious about being abstinent from opiates after all these years.

Helen's stepfather was killed in a motor vehicle accident when she was ten years of age. She was in the vehicle at the time. At that time, her parents were in the process of separating. Helen saw a psychiatrist at the age of twelve or thirteen when she was asked to leave home by her mother due to her defiant behaviour. She subsequently entered foster care, which she left permanently at the age of sixteen. She suffered various forms of physical and sexual abuse before moving out on her own.

Helen had a Grade 10 education. She described her ten-year marriage as very positive, and her ex-husband as supportive. On one occasion, she had been given a prescription for antidepressants, but never filled it; she did not see herself-as depressed or particularly anxious. She acknowledged feeling unhappy but attributed this to her addiction and life struggles. She had cut her wrists in her early teens but had no other suicidal thoughts or attempts and had not cut herself-for years. There was no history of eating disorder.

Helen did not know her biological father's family history. She did know that she had alcoholic uncles. She was not aware of any mental illness or suicides in the family.

The initial interview and assessment. During our initial interview, she was extremely critical of her methadone-prescribing physician, whom she alleged was "in it for the money and had thousands of patients." The physician had apparently not monitored her thirty-year use of methadone, or monitored her for any other opiate medications or other classes of drug. She had continued to be an active heroin user throughout her using career. Presumably through her intravenous drug use, she was diagnosed with hepatitis C in the mid-1980s, for which she had received no treatment. Most methadone-prescribing physicians these days would likely have considered her dosage of 50 to 70 mg to be too low, and would have increased her dosage, given her ongoing active use of heroin.

Helen was a drug addict with an extensive history of abuse, abandonment, and neglect; not an unfamiliar history for drug addicts. Equally striking, however, was her remarkable resilience. In spite of her chronic addiction, poor physical health, and obviously very difficult upbringing, she was delightful and engaging, had a positive attitude, and exhibited a wonderful sense of humour. In many ways, she had done extremely well, maintaining her employment for the last eighteen years.

Helen could easily have been described as precontemplative in the stages of change model at the time of her employer's intervention. She had resigned herself-to chronic opiate addiction, in spite of her awareness of the negative consequences of her ongoing issues. She appreciated the care expressed by her employer and was willing to take advantage of the opportunity.

In terms of the ASAM criteria for the six dimensions of multidimensional assessment (see chapter 7, Detoxification) and clinical placement setting for treatment, she was clearly an appropriate candidate for intensive residential treatment.

Dimension 1: Helen required medical management of her opiate withdrawal, given the duration of her use, the quantity she used, and her intravenous route of administration.

Dimension 2: Helen had a diagnosis of hepatitis C and chronic obstructive pulmonary disease, otherwise being reasonably stable medically.

Dimension 3: Helen had experienced considerable turbulence and chaos in her early childhood and adolescence. There were no significant concurrent psychiatric disorders.

Dimension 4: Helen came into treatment through an intervention by her employer. At that time she was precontemplative. She valued her job and agreed to come into residential treatment as a requirement of employment.

Dimension 5: Helen had been continuously using opiates intravenously for a few decades, with no significant periods of abstinence. Her risk for relapse and continued use was felt to be extremely high.

Dimension 6: Helen lived alone. She was not in a relationship. She tended to isolate herself-from others and her family system was dysfunctional. This also placed her in a high-risk category.

Under the DSM IV-TR, her diagnosis would clearly be opiate dependence. Her DSM-5 diagnosis was opiate use disorder–severe.

Helen's treatment. Helen was started on Suboxone with an initial test dose of 4 mg followed by a subsequent 8 mg dose later on the first day. Her opiate withdrawal symptoms settled and 12 mg was her maximal dose. This was gradually tapered, with a dose reduction every two days. Toward the end of the tapering period, her opiate withdrawal scales began to increase and she began to experience active symptoms of opiate withdrawal. The latter portion of her Suboxone taper was restarted and a subsequent review of her COWS results showed that she was comfortable; she managed the rest of her detoxification well.

She was prescribed Gabapentin 600 mg three times daily as needed and 600 to 900 mg for insomnia as needed. Insomnia remained problematic and Trazodone 50 to 100 mg was added. The Gabapentin was extremely helpful for management of her anxiety, insomnia, muscle twitching, and restlessness.

Identified medical issues included the fact that she was positive for hepatitis C, had lost considerable weight, and had chronic obstructive pulmonary disease. Psychiatric assessment did not identify any concurrent psychiatric disorder, although she clearly had an extensive history of abuse, neglect, and early childhood chaos.

Helen initially expressed feelings of low self-esteem and confidence. Complex issues arising from childhood often make group therapy challenging, as it requires a level of intimacy and trust in others. However, Helen was able to actively engage and open up in group therapy. In spite of being relatively open in group, she found it difficult to socialize, but this gradually improved throughout her treatment. She presented as very motivated and keen to discover her "real self." She was highly motivated in completing her assignments, and had no problem accepting that she was an addict and acknowledging that she had the disease of addiction. In response to the question on one of her assignments, "What crises besides the one that got you into treatment now would have eventually happened?" she responded: "I would have died. . . . I was slowly killing myself."

Helen completed the inpatient phase of residential treatment. She was advised to continue in the extended treatment program, based on her continued treatment need, chronicity, severity of use, and limited social supports. She agreed to this and continued to actively participate in treatment.

JAKE

Jake was a gay professional in his late forties. Previously, he had been in several committed, relatively short-term, relationships, all with male partners. He was admitted for residential treatment of alcohol dependence, as well as a six-year period of abuse of cocaine and methamphetamine, typically associated with sexual behaviours.

Before treatment. Jake started drinking at the age of twelve. He drank on weekends, excessively, during his twenties. His drinking escalated further throughout his thirties, when he drank on an almost daily basis with his partner at the time. His drinking took a major jump after the relationship ended. For the last six years, he estimated he now drank a bottle of wine daily, as well as binge drinking much more heavily a couple of times a month. On these occasions he also used cocaine or methamphetamine and engaged in excessive sexual behaviours. He estimated his cocaine use was once or twice monthly, approximately 1 g per occasion. This always started with drinking first, followed by cocaine use, then by sexual behaviours. He had also used GHB at these times.

Jake had a lengthy history of sexually addictive behaviours beginning in his early twenties. This initially started with cruising in parks and public bathrooms, which progressed to various other locations including public facilities, fitness centres, bathhouses, and sex clubs; eventually, he began hiring prostitutes. He noticed a progressive increase in the frequency and risk associated with these behaviours. More recently he had engaged in online cruising, online sex chat, and using the Internet to make live connections. He had been diagnosed with HIV approximately five years previously, but this did not significantly change his sexual behaviour.

Jake had experienced alcohol-induced blackouts and alcohol withdrawal symptoms. His driver's licence had twice been suspended for twenty-four-hours, but he still drank and drove on a number of occasions. His addiction had had a negative impact on the quality of his work; at times he was unable to work. His relationships had clearly been negatively impacted. He had had some supportive counselling but had not had any residential treatment.

Jake described distinct episodes of major depression beginning in his twenties. His depressive symptoms were typical; generally, he had had a positive response to antidepressant medication although he was currently taking antidepressants with only a partially positive response. He had attempted suicide many years previously and currently occasionally experienced vague suicidal thoughts. He also described a lengthy history of anxiety.

Jake said his mother was an alcoholic who also suffered from depression. There were apparently many alcoholic relatives on his mother's side of the family.

Jake's case suggested the probability of an independent primary mood disorder (see chapter 9, Concurrent Disorders). From the history we obtained, we saw that Jake suffered classic depressive symptoms which responded completely and robustly to antidepressant medications. Previous attempts to discontinue medication led to relapse of depression. There was a strong seasonal element to the depression with no history of hypomanic or manic behaviours. The sexual behaviours were a relatively constant feature and did not fluctuate specifically with mood, which might otherwise have indicated manic symptoms. Of interest was the observation that the patient's mother suffered from both addiction and depression.

Jake's case raises the complex issues and relationships between addiction and sexuality. This is a very important area in addiction. (See chapter 4, Sexuality and Addiction, for a discussion of this relationship.)

Jake's treatment. Jake was admitted for residential treatment of his addiction, after unsuccessful attempts to manage it using outpatient approaches. He did not require detoxification. He completed a medical and psychiatric assessment on admission and was diagnosed with alcohol dependence as well as cocaine, methamphetamine, and GHB abuse, according to DSM IV-TR criteria. He was also diagnosed with major depressive disorder and generalized anxiety disorder and was noted to be HIV-positive. He was receiving appropriate treatment for this from a specialist.

Since he was medically stable, his initial treatment focused on addiction and mental health issues. Throughout the course of treatment, Jake continued to express concern regarding his ongoing symptoms of depression, which in the past had normally responded well to treatment. We made appropriate changes to his antidepressant medication. At the time of completing treatment, Jake noted that his mood was somewhat better; however, he still felt moderate depressive symptoms, in spite of now being on a combination of three different antidepressants.

Jake described some initial difficulties engaging in treatment. In spite of being very intelligent and articulate, he found group situations to be very intimidating. He had been bullied in the past and witnessed violence toward other gay men, making him extremely anxious around the more dominant males ("rednecks") who were in treatment. He had significant difficulty in trusting others and was fearful of judgment and intimidation. In spite of these initial fears, he was able to open up in group and did not experience any of the problems that he had anticipated.

Counselling staff identified and thoroughly reviewed his sexually addictive behaviours. His significant issues of guilt and shame were compounded by this addictive behaviour. However, he was able to share this aspect of his addiction selectively, with trusted male peers. He found this very difficult but also experienced relief.

At times it was difficult for him to connect with his emotions, which he had been used to repressing, using his intellect instead. Gradually, he was able to increase his access to feelings and communicate these to others. He tended to rely heavily on his own opinion, and was reluctant to accept feedback from others. He had a tendency to filter out the positive, seeing only the negative in himself. His cognitive style was quite self-defeating and efforts were made to help him with his appraisal. He had difficulties accepting the disease model of alcoholism and tended to see himself as a personal failure. Passive-aggressive tendencies were identified. People noticed that he tended to slip into a victim mode, in which he engaged in self-pity. He tended to be a perfectionist, and could easily be self-critical and critical of those around him. As a psychiatrist, one of my clinical challenges was to try and tease out his addiction dynamics from his depressive symptoms. Many of the factors identified above reflected relatively stable traits as opposed to mood-related traits.

Jake committed to a set of aftercare recommendations that included attending three or four twelve-step meetings weekly, attending aftercare appointments weekly, obtaining a temporary sponsor within one week of leaving treatment, and calling the sponsor once weekly. He committed to calling someone in recovery three or four times weekly, to reinforce reaching out and getting support from others, which was always difficult for him. He also agreed to having a home group within two weeks of leaving, and to eating three meals daily, reading recovery material, and taking appropriate medications. The medical team communicated current medical issues regarding depression, anxiety, and HIV with his attending family doctor. Medication updates were provided.

Jake initially struggled after leaving treatment. He apparently relapsed in terms of sexual behaviours which in turn led to relapsing to chemicals. He was able to use the relapse as a wake-up call and subsequently tightened up his recovery behaviours. He has since made significant gains.

HANK

Hank, sixty-two years old, had been with his current partner for almost ten years; before that he had been married for twelve years. His children were in their twenties. He had retired several years previously, after suffering a head injury in a motor vehicle accident. He had been in a coma for approximately one week after the accident. He felt there were no long-term consequences from the injury.

Hank was pressured into treatment. "I have a couple of difficult relatives," he said. He significantly minimized the extent of his drinking. He did admit to drinking "twenty-six ounces a day of hard liquor for the last three years," but collateral information suggested that this was closer to forty ounces daily for the last five or six years. He admitted to experiencing blackouts. He also noted having withdrawal symptoms in the morning for which he required alcohol. His activities had been dramatically reduced outside the home and his social life was significantly restricted.

He would begin drinking first thing in the morning. He had a seizure one year previously, while in a detoxification program at a hospital. He immediately returned to drinking after leaving the hospital. Recently, he had been charged with impaired driving. His partner was concerned about his drinking. He had not made any attempts to quit, and had had no prior treatment for addiction.

He was admitted for residential treatment of his alcohol dependence. However, he stated that he planned to leave after a few days and "become a moderate drinker like my father." He also had been a daily smoker for years. He had no significant psychiatric history. Hank described three maternal uncles and a son who are alcoholic. He had recently been worried about his son who was currently receiving treatment for his alcoholism. He was not aware of any family history of mental illness.

Hank's treatment. Hank had an obvious diagnosis of alcohol dependence under DSM IV-TR, or alcohol use disorder–severe using DSM-5 criteria.

According to the ASAM criteria he was an appropriate candidate for level 3.5, Clinically Managed High-Intensity Residential Services:

Dimension 1: Hank was a daily heavy drinker with a history of significant alcohol withdrawal and withdrawal seizures in the past. He would require medication-assisted detoxification in a supervised setting.

Dimension 2:   He had a history of alcohol withdrawal seizures; otherwise, he was reasonably stable medically.

Dimension 3:   Hank had no psychiatric illness. His previous head injury may possibly have caused cognitive impairment, but limited information was available on this.

Dimension 4:   Hank was precontemplative to contemplative. He had no interest in abstaining from alcohol and had presented himself-for treatment on the basis of ultimatums from family. He was clear from the outset that he had no intentions of completing treatment, and wanted to become "a social drinker like my father."

Dimension 5:   Hank had a high level of risk for relapse or continued use. He had advanced denial, minimal motivation, and had no interest in abstaining from alcohol. The probability of "social drinking" as he described it was minimal.

Dimension 6:   Hank's family was fed up with his drinking and had run out of patience.

Hank was clearly a risk for alcohol withdrawal. On the basis of his daily heavy drinking for several years, combined with the fact that he had previous alcohol withdrawal seizures, he was placed on a heavy lorazepam detoxification regime. He was started on lorazepam 2 mg three times daily and 1 mg at bedtime. This was tapered over the following six days. Review of his CIWA withdrawal scores and clinical status demonstrated that he was comfortable on this program.

Laboratory result analysis demonstrated significantly elevated liver enzymes including GGT of 182 (normal is less than 58), AST 306 (normal is less than 35), ALT 238 (normal is less than 60) and total bilirubin 37 (normal is less than 20; note, elevated bilirubin causes jaundice, and yellowing of the skin or whites of the eyes can be seen).

Once Hank was detoxified from alcohol, he insisted on leaving treatment. Counsellors spent considerable time encouraging him to remain in treatment. Several patients in treatment also attempted to talk him into remaining. When these approaches failed, an emergency family conference took place. In spite of all of these efforts, Hank left treatment against medical advice. No follow-up was available for the case, but his prognosis was obviously poor.

Epilogue

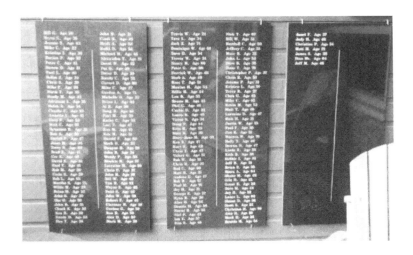

This plaque is mounted at the entry of Edgewood. The 177 names engraved on it belong to men and women who completed treatment, relapsed to their drug of choice – and died. It is a harsh reminder that addictions kill people.

Everyone on this list had a social network of family members – spouses, partners, parents, grandparents, brothers and sisters , children, friends, coworkers. Their deaths reverberated throughout these networks, affecting everyone. As treatment providers who have put their hearts and souls into working with patients during their treatment, we too experience a strong sense of loss when any of our patients die from the disease. Staff are always moved to tears when patients walk out of treatment in a bad state of mind, because they know how likely it is that those patients will return to using alcohol or drugs, and that they might die as a result.

Addiction is about unbearable pain and loss. But it is also about unnecessary tragedy, because this is a *treatable* disease. Edgewood has a monthly Cake Night, where alumni are invited to return and celebrate various landmarks in their recovery, ranging from thirty days to decades, and staff celebrate these accomplishments with them. These are the miracles of recovery. Their lives have been entirely transformed. Many of these patients had presented in very rough shape at the time of their admission — severely affected by their addiction and so hopeless that they were seriously contemplating suicide. As they share their stories, many recognize that they had been on the brink of dying. They are often accompanied by family members who struggled with the pain of not knowing whether their loved one would live or die in the next twenty-four hours. The gratitude is palpable. These are the moments that make all of the rigours of providing treatment worthwhile. And Cake Night always contains surprises. I have long given up trying to guess who will do well in recovery, and who won't. Some of the most refractory patients have done extremely well, and those who seem to have had the best chance relapsed almost immediately.

Many addiction writers who oppose the twelve-step process find the concept of powerlessness offensive. They say that they want to empower people, not leave them in their powerlessness. But one of the common themes of successful recovery is surrender. Somehow, a striking paradox emerges: when people acknowledge their powerlessness, they become empowered. When they truly and deeply understand that returning to their substance of choice is not an option, and when they follow the aftercare plan faithfully, they get there. Empowerment results, an empowerment based on a new rationality.

Alcohol and drugs are not essential nutrients, and the risks of returning to alcohol and drug use are immense. In the past, patients may have thought they could return to a behaviour that had so many negative consequences for them, and hope for a better outcome or a controlled use. Now, they deeply know the irrationality of this, and their minds are freed. They can make a full commitment to moving ahead with abstinence and recovery.

In closing, several thoughts come to my mind.

First and foremost, it is my hope that this book will be interesting and useful for people suffering from substance use disorders or addiction, and their families. My goal was also to provide a helpful and up-to-date resource for their caregivers.

Although I work in a twelve-step facilitation setting, I wanted to communicate a respectful appreciation in this book for the many philosophies and orientations of treatment out there. I have been very impressed by the creativity of thought and the different approaches taken to improve the lives of individuals suffering from addiction. I always reflect on the fact that addiction disorders and patients are wide ranging, and require a variety of different approaches. As I have noted, existing long-term outcome research is limited. It is clearly needed, to direct future treatment and improve success rates. All approaches make their contribution, and mutual respect and cooperation is needed. Whatever the philosophy or approach, I am humbled to observe that addiction workers are unified in their passion to help those suffering from addiction.

I am concerned about the diminishing resources available for withdrawal management and intensive treatment on the more severe end of the continuum. The demand for these resources is likely to continue to expand, particularly given the trend toward escalating opiate dependence.

However, I am encouraged to see the growth of addiction medicine and addiction psychiatry in Canada. We have been blessed with several strong leaders in this field in the past, and many very talented physicians are entering this area of specialization. I believe that an expanded interest in the area of addiction and occupational medicine will lead to better recognition of the problem of addiction, and the opportunity for those employees who are suffering from substance use disorders to receive the treatment that they require.

It will be very interesting to see where the medical marijuana issue takes us over the next several years.

In conclusion, I would like to thank Edgewood for giving me the opportunity and support required to write this book. I have found treating patients with addictions to be a highly rewarding area of medicine. I would strongly encourage any health professional with an interest in this area to explore opportunities for education and training, and consider a career in addictions.

Acknowledgments

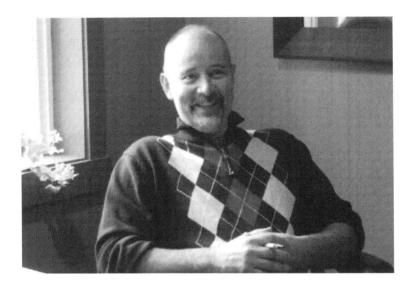

Dr. Merville Vincent

First and foremost, I have been very blessed: I was raised in a household full of joy, love, and laughter. While I may have taken this somewhat for granted during my childhood, I have increasingly recognized what an amazing gift this was. Without it, I almost certainly would not have had the confidence or opportunity to work as a psychiatrist in this field. In particular, I would like to thank my father for being the ultimate role model as an addiction psychiatrist, wonderful father, and special human being. My mother was kind enough to pass on her compassion, sensitivity and listening skills. My brothers always brought joy and companionship over the years.

I have had several highly valued role models in the various treatment settings I have worked in. It has been a pleasure to work with so many amazing counsellors, nursing staff, and various other employees, particularly at Edgewood. Working at Edgewood has been a continuous learning experience. I have never seen such passion and dedication as I have experienced there.

I sincerely appreciate the gracious support of Edgewood throughout the process of writing this book. I would like to give a special thank-you to Lorne Hildebrand, Rochelle Hildebrand, Dr. Charlie Whelton, Lis Muise, and Elizabeth Loudon, for their valuable feedback throughout this process. The generous support from the library staff at the College of Physicians and Surgeons of BC has also been greatly appreciated over the years.

Dr. Graeme Cunningham, a unique mentor to me throughout my work in addiction medicine, deserves special mention. I have learned so much from him and have always placed a great value on our relationship.

I was fortunate enough to find my beautiful wife Deb at the early age of eighteen! We will have just celebrated thirty-five years of marriage by the time this book is published. I guess in this case I am "addicted to love"! Our lives have been enriched by the addition of our three children: Michael, Laura, and Rebecca, who have brought us great joy and continual entertainment.

Lastly, my greatest teachers have been the patients who have struggled to rebuild their lives following the often devastating effects of addiction. I have marvelled at their courage and resilience. I have been humbled by their willingness to open up and share the most intimate of secrets, where previous life lessons had taught them to trust no one. I have repeatedly had the opportunity to share the joy of a life reclaimed and a family restored. My hope is that this book may in some way help to reduce suffering from addiction.

Glossary

AA. Alcoholics Anonymous.

acamprosate. Marketed as Campral, a medication to aid in abstinence from alcohol.

ADD, ADHD. Attention deficit disorder, attention deficit and hyperactivity disorder.

Advil (ibuprofen). A nonsteroidal anti-inflammatory drug (NSAID).

alprazolam. Marketed as Xanax. A benzodiazepine.

Ambien (zolpidem). A sleeping pill. One of the "Z" drugs.

Antabuse. Brand name of disulfiram, a drug used to treat alcohol dependence.

ASAM. American Society of Addiction Medicine.

Ativan (lorazepam). A benzodiazepine, generally used to treat anxiety and insomnia.

atomoxetine. Marketed as Strattera. A nonaddictive medication used for treating ADD/ADHD.

barbiturate. A central nervous system depressant.

"bath salts." A stimulant street drug.

benzodiazepines. Drugs with sedative properties, used in the management of anxiety. Marketed as Valium, Librium, and others. These drugs have a tendency to cause tolerance, physical dependence, and withdrawal symptoms upon cessation after long-term use.

buprenorphine. A semisynthetic opioid, used to treat opioid addiction and in the management of pain.

bupropion. Marketed as Zyban (for smoking cessation) and Wellbutrin (as an antidepressant).

CADDRA. Canadian ADHD Resource Alliance.

Campral. Brand name of acamprosate, a medication to aid in abstinence from alcohol.

cathinones. Drugs in the amphetamine family. The parent compound cathinone is found in khat. Synthetic cathinones abused include mephadrone and methylone.

chlordiazepoxide (Librium). A long-acting benzodiazepine.

Cipralex (escitalopram). An SSRI antidepressant.

clonazepam. Marketed as Rivotril. A long-acting benzodiazepine.

clonidine. An antihypertensive medication also commonly used in the treatment of withdrawal from opiates.

cross addiction. The elevated risk of becoming addicted to other substances than one is originally addicted to.

Cymbalta. Brand name of duloxetine. An SNRI antidepressant.

Dexedrine (dextroamphetamine). A stimulant widely prescribed by physicians for the treatment of ADHD.

diazepam. Valium.

Dilaudid. Brand name of hydromorphone. A pain reliever.

disulfiram. Marketed as Antabuse. A drug used to treat alcohol dependence.

divalproex. An anticonvulsant medication for treatment of seizure disorders, also used as a treatment for bipolar disorder.

dopamine. A neurochemical that mediates pleasurable experience, reinforcing behaviours that promote human adaptation as a species — sexual, eating, social, and other functions.

DSM-5. The *Diagnostic and Statistical Manual of Mental Disorders,* 5th edition.

DTs (delirium tremens). A clinical syndrome characterized by disorientation to person, place, and time as well as confusion and possible hallucinations. DTs are a complication of advanced alcohol dependence, typically occurring a few days after abrupt discontinuation of alcohol consumption.

duloxetine. An antidepressant marketed as Cymbalta.

DXM (dextromethorphan). A cough suppressant that can also act as a dissociative hallucinogen.

Ecstasy. A street drug with hallucinogenic and stimulant properties; MDMA in the pure form. but often adulterated in community samples.

Effexor. Brand name of venlafaxine. An SNRI antidepressant.

EMDR. Eye movement desensitization and reprocessing. A specific treatment for PTSD.

endorphin. An opiate produced by the body.

fentanyl. A synthetic opioid, 50 to 100 times more potent than morphine on a dose-by-dose basis.

Fiorinal. A combination medication used to manage migraine headaches.

FIRST. Acronym: For Inspiration and Recognition of Science and Technology.

GABA (gamma-aminobutyric) receptor. A chemical messenger in the brain which reduces the activity of the neurons to which it binds.

Gabapentin. An anticonvulsant medication with off-indication uses in the treatment of neuropathic pain and anxiety/insomnia.

GHB (gamma hydroxybutyrate). A sedative substance, similar in effect to alcohol. Also known as the "date rape" drug.

glutamate. Also known as glutamic acid, this amino acid neurotransmitter is a key player in learning and memory.

Gravol. A drug used to prevent nausea and vomiting.

high. Experience of euphoria, from a drug or behaviour.

hydromorphone. A synthetic opioid, used as a pain reliever.

ibuprofen (Advil). A nonsteroidal anti-inflammatory drug (NSAID).

Imovane (zopiclone). A sleeping pill. One of the "Z" drugs.

ketamine. A veterinary anesthetic agent; a common drug of abuse.

kindling. A process whereby a brain event is both initiated and its recurrence is made more likely. In substance withdrawal, the condition that results from repeated withdrawal episodes from either alcohol or benzodiazepines, where each withdrawal experience leads to more severe withdrawal symptoms than the previous withdrawal syndrome.

K2. A synthetic cannabinoid. Also known as Spice and many other names.

Librium (chlordiazepoxide). A long-acting benzodiazepine.

lorazepam. Ativan.

Maxeran. An antiemetic drug.

MDMA. The pure form of Ecstasy.

methadone. A synthetic opioid, used to treat addiction to other opioid drugs, including heroin and oxycodone. Also used to manage pain.

mirtazapine. A tetracyclic antidepressant. Also called Remeron.

NA. Narcotics Anonymous.

naltrexone. An opiate antagonist or blocker. Also marketed as Revia, used to reduce alcohol dependence.

neuroadaptation. A process whereby the nervous system makes adaptive changes in an attempt to maintain normalcy in response to repeated drug use.

NIAAA. National Institute on Alcohol Abuse and Alcoholism, part of the U.S. National Institutes of Health (NIH).

NSAID. Nonsteroidal anti-inflammatory drug.

OxyContin. A long-acting form of oxycodone.

oxycodone. An opiate medication, available in short- or long-acting formulations.

OxyNEO. A long-acting formulation of oxycodone, less amenable to tampering than OxyContin.

paroxetine (trade name Paxil). An SSRI antidepressant.

Paxil (paroxetine). An SSRI antidepressant.

Percocet. A pain reliever containing short-acting oxycodone and acetaminophen.

PCP (phencyclidine). Also known as *angel dust.* A stimulant drug of abuse.

prazosin. An alpha-blocker. Used in the treatment of PTSD.

propanolol. A beta-blocker. Marketed as Inderal. Typically used for treatment of hypertension, but also for some forms of anxiety.

PTSD. Posttraumatic stress disorder.

quetiapine. An atypical antipsychotic; marketed as Seroquel.

Revia. Brand name of naltrexone, a medication used in alcohol reduction.

Ritalin (methylphenidate). A central nervous system stimulant, typically used for treatment of ADD/ADHD.

Rivotril (clonazepam). A long-acting benzodiazepine, generally used to treat anxiety and insomnia.

SAMHSA. Substance Abuse and Mental Health Services Administration.

sensitization. A neurological process that occurs more easily or rapidly with repeated experience.

SNRI. Serotonin-norepinephrine reuptake inhibitor. Antidepressant drug. Examples include Effexor and Cymbalta.

SSRI. Selective serotonin uptake inhibitor. A family of antidepressant medications.

Spice. A synthetic cannabinoid. Also known as K2 and many other names.

Suboxone. A drug combining buprenorphine and naloxone, used to treat withdrawal from opiates and for maintenance treatment of opiate addiction, similar to the use of methadone.

Temposil. Causes aversive symptoms when alcohol is ingested; similar to Antabuse.

THC (tetrahydrocannabinol). The active ingredient in marijuana.

thiamine. Vitamin B1.

tolerance. More substance needed to generate the same effect.

Topamax. Brand name of topiramate, an anticonvulsant, studied for its potential benefit in treatment relapse in alcoholics.

topiramate. Marketed as Topamax. An anticonvulsant, studied for its potential benefit in treatment relapse in alcoholics.

Trazodone. A tetracyclic antidepressant, typically used for treatment of insomnia.

tricyclics. A family of antidepressants first used in the 1950s. Largely replaced by SSRIs and SNRIs.

Valium (diazepam). A benzodiazepine, generally used to treat anxiety and insomnia.

varenicline. A smoking cessation drug, marketed in Canada as Champix and in the United States as Chantix.

venlafaxine. An antidepressant marketed as Effexor.

Wellbutrin. Brand name of bupropion (used as an antidepressant).

Xanax (alprazolam). A benzodiazepine, generally used to treat anxiety and insomnia.

"Z" drugs. Nonbenzodiazepine drugs used for insomnia. Zolpidem (Ambien) and zopiclone (Imovane) are two main examples.

zolpidem. Marketed as Ambien. A medication used for insomnia.

zopiclone. Marketed as Imovane. A medication used for insomnia.

Zyban. Brand name of bupropion (used for smoking cessation).

Further Reading

Note: The abbreviation "n.d." indicates that no date was available for the publication or online source.

Alcohol abuse, eating disorders share genetic link. 2013. *ScienceDaily*. August 21. http://www.sciencedaily.com/releases/2013/08/130821084832.htm (accessed May 26, 2014).

Alcoholics Anonymous. 2006. *Alcoholics Anonymous big book*. [S. I.]: BN Pub.

Alexander, Bruce K. n.d. *Addiction: The view from Rat Park*. http://globalizationofaddiction.ca/articles-speeches/148-addiction-the-view-from-rat-park.html (accessed May 25, 2014).

American Psychiatric Association. 2013. *Diagnostic and statistical manual of mental disorders*. 5th ed. Arlington, VA: American Psychiatric Publishing.

Anderson, Pauline. 2014. *Teen marijuana use linked to earlier psychosis onset* (from the American Psychiatric Association's 2014 Annual Meeting). *Medscape Medical News*. May 14. http://www.medscape .com/viewarticle/825131 (accessed June 30, 2014).

Ashton, C. Heather. 2002. *Benzodiazepines: How they work and how to withdraw (aka The Ashton Manual)*. http://www.benzo.org.uk/manual /contents.htm (accessed May 26, 2014).

Atheist alcoholics seek to be well without "God." 2014. *The Vancouver Sun*. April 5. http://blogs.vancouversun.com/2014/04/05/atheist-alcoholics-finding-recovery-without-the-god-talk (accessed May 25, 2014).

Beck, Aaron T., Fred D. Wright, Cory F. Newman, and Bruce S. Liese. 1993. *Cognitive therapy of substance abuse*. New York, NY: The Guilford Press.

Benedek, David D., Matthew J. Friedman, Douglas Zatzick, and Robert J. Ursano. 2009. Guideline watch (March 2009): Practice guideline for the treatment of patients with acute stress disorder and posttraumatic stress disorder. *Psychiatry Online*. doi: 10.1176/appi.books.9780890423479 .156498 (accessed May 26, 2014).

Biernacki, Patrick. 1986. *Pathways from heroin addiction: Recovery without treatment.* Philadelphia, PA: Temple University Press.

Bisson, Jonathan I., and Andrew M. 2005. Psychological treatment of post-traumatic stress disorder (PTSD). *Cochrane Database of Systematic Reviews* April 18, no. 2: CD003388. http://www.ncbi.nlm.nih.gov/pubmed /17636720 (accessed May 26, 2014).

———. 2007. Psychological treatment of post-traumatic stress disorder (PTSD). *Cochrane Database of Systematic Reviews* July 18, no. 3: CD003388. http://www.ncbi.nlm.nih.gov/pubmed/17636720 (accessed May 26, 2014).

Bisson, Jonathan I., N. P. Roberts, Andrew M., Cooper R., and Lewis C. 2013. Psychological therapies for chronic post-traumatic stress disorder (PTSD) in adults. *Cochrane Database System Reviews*, no. 12: CD003388. doi: 10.1002/14651858.CD003388.pub4 (accessed July 4, 2014).

British Columbia Coroners Service. 2013. *Opiate deaths.* http://www.pssg .gov.bc.ca/coroners/reports/docs/OpiateDeaths.pdf (accessed May 26, 2014).

British Columbia Ministry of Health. 2013. *Problem drinking.* http://www.bcguidelines.ca/guideline_problem_drinking.html (accessed May 26, 2014).

Brooks, Megan 2014. Opioid addiction meds effective but buprenorphine a better bet? *Psychiatric Services* 65: 146–70. http://www.medscape .com/viewarticle/820893 (accessed June 26, 2014).

Brown, Sandra, and Marc Schuckit. 1988. Changes in depression among abstinent alcoholics. *Journal of Studies on Alcohol and Drugs* 49: 412–7.

CAGE questionnaire. n.d. http://www.integration.samhsa.gov/clinical-practice/sbirt/CAGE_questionaire.pdf (accessed June 21, 22014).

Canadian ADHD Resource Alliance (CADDRA). 2010. *Canadian ADHD practice guidelines (CAP-guidelines)* (3rd ed.). http://www.caddra.ca/pdfs /caddraGuidelines2011.pdf (accessed May 25, 2014).

Canadian Psychiatric Association. 2006. Clinical practice guidelines: Management of anxiety disorders. *The Canadian Journal of Psychiatry* 51, no. 8, Supp. 2 (July). http://publications.cpa-apc.org/media .php?mid=451 (accessed May 25, 2014).

Canadian Human Rights Commission. 2009. *Canadian Human Rights Commission's policy on alcohol and drug testing.* http://www.chrc-ccdp.gc.ca/sites/default/files/padt_pdda_eng.pdf (accessed May 26, 2014).

Carnes, Patrick J. 2001. *Out of the shadows: Understanding sexual addiction.* Center City, MN: Hazelden.

Carnes, Patrick J., and Kenneth M. Adams. 2002. *Clinical management of sex addiction.* New York, NY: Brunner-Routledge.

Carnes, Patrick J., David L. Delmonico, and Elizabeth Griffin. 2001. *In the shadows of the net: Breaking free of compulsive online sexual behavior.* Center City, MN: Hazelden.

Centers for Disease Control and Prevention (CDC). 2013. *Opioids drive continued increase in drug overdose deaths.* http://www.cdc.gov /media/releases/2013/p0220_drug_overdose_deaths.html (accessed May 26, 2014).

———. 2014. *Physicians are a leading source of prescription opioids for the highest-risk users.* http://www.cdc.gov/media/releases/2014/p0303-prescription-opioids.html (accessed May 26, 2014).

———. 2014. *Prescription drug overdose in the United States: Fact sheet.* http://www.cdc.gov/homeandrecreationalsafety/overdose/facts.html (accessed May 26, 2014).

Centre for Addiction and Mental Health (CAMH). n.d. *What are concurrent disorders?* http://www.camh.ca/en/hospital/health_information /a_z_mental_health_and_addiction_information/concurrent_disorders/ concurrent_substance_use_and_mental_health_disorders_information_g uide/Pages/what_are_cd_infoguide.aspx#notes (accessed May 26, 2014).

————. 2001. Clinical institute withdrawal assessment for alcohol (CIWA). http://www.reseaufranco.com/en/assessment_and_treatment _information/assessment_tools/clinical_institute_withdrawal_assessme nt_for_alcohol_ciwa.pdf (accessed June 23, 2014).

Chang, L. C., S. R. Raty, J. Ortiz, N. S. Bailard, and S. J. Mathew. 2013. The emerging use of ketamine for anesthesia and sedation in traumatic brain injuries. [Special issue: Ketamine revisited]. *CNS Neuroscience & Therapeutics* 19, no. 6: 390–5. doi: 10.1111/cns.12077 (accessed June 19, 2014).

Chengappa, Kn Roy, Joseph Levine, Samuel Gershon, and David J. Kupfer. 2008. Lifetime prevalence of substance or alcohol abuse and dependence among subjects with bipolar I and II disorders in a voluntary registry. *Bipolar Disorders* 2, no. 3: 191–5. doi: 10.1034/j.1399-5618.2000.020306.x (accessed May 25, 2014).

Clinical Opiate Withdrawal Scale (COWS). n.d. www.emcdda.europa .eu/attachements.cfm/att_35646_EN_COWS.pdf (accessed June 24, 2014).

Dale, Lowell. 2014. *What are electronic cigarettes? Are they safer than conventional cigarettes?* http://www.mayoclinic.org/healthy-living/quit-smoking/expert-answers/electronic-cigarettes/faq-20057776 (accessed May 26, 2014).

Davis, Caroline. 2013. From passive overeating to "food addiction": A spectrum of compulsion and severity. *ISRN Obesity* 2013, Article ID 435027. doi: http://dx.doi.org/10.1155/2013/435027 (accessed May 26, 2014).

Del Re, A. C., Adam J. Gordon, Anna Lembke, and Alex H. S. Harris. 2013. Prescription of topiramate to treat alcohol use disorders in the Veterans Health Administration. *Addiction Science & Clinical Practice* 8, no. 12. doi: 10.1186/1940-0640-8-12 (accessed May 26, 2014).

Derrick, Chad. 2013. A dangerous hallucinogenic drug—easily and legally available. *CTV W5*. March 2. http://www.ctvnews.ca/w5/a-dangerous-hallucinogenic-drug-easily-and-legally-available-1.1178395 (accessed May 25, 2014).

DiClemente, Carlo C. 2003. *Addiction and change: How addictions develop and addicted people recover*. New York, NY: The Guilford Press.

Dimeff, Linda A., and Marsha M. Linehan. 2008. Dialectical behavior therapy for substance abusers. *Addiction Science & Clinical Practice* 4, no. 2: 39–47. http://www.ncbi.nlm.nih.gov/pmc/articles/PMC2797106 (accessed May 26, 2014).

Dole, Vincent P., and Marie E. Nyswander. 1965. A medical treatment for diacetylmorphine (heroin) addiction: A clinical trial with methadone hydrochloride. *JAMA* 193, no. 8: 646–50. doi: 10.1001/jama.1965 .03090080008002 (accessed May 26, 2014).

Dutra, Lauren M., and Stanton A. Glantz. 2014. Electronic cigarettes and conventional cigarette use among US adolescents: A cross-sectional study. *JAMA Pediatrics* (March 6). doi: 10.1001/jamapediatrics.2013.5488 (accessed May 26, 2014).

Fantegrossi, William E., Jeffery H. Moran, Anna Radominska-Pandya, and Paul Prather. 2014. Distinct pharmacology and metabolism of K2 synthetic cannabinoids compared to Δ(9)-THC: Mechanism underlying greater toxicity? *Life Sciences* 97, no. 1: 45–54. doi: 10.1016/j.lfs.2013 .09.017 (accessed May 26, 2014).

Feder, Adriana, Michael Parides, James W. Murrough, Andrew M. Perez, Julia E. Morgan, Shireen Saxena, Katherine Kirkwood, Marije aan het Rot, Kyle Lapidus, Le-Ben Wan, Dan Iosifescu, and Dennis S. Charney. 2014. Efficacy of intravenous ketamine for treatment of chronic posttraumatic stress disorder: A randomized clinical trial. *JAMA Psychiatry* (April 16). doi: 10.1001/jamapsychiatry.2014.62 (accessed May 25, 2014).

Fiscella, Kevin. 2012. Buprenorphine maintenance therapy in opioid-addicted health care professionals returning to clinical practice. *Mayo Clinic Proceedings* 87, no. 8 (March): 806. doi: http://dx.doi.org/10.1016 /j.mayocp.2012.04.008 (accessed May 25, 2014).

Foa, Edna B., and Terence M. Keane. 2008. *Effective treatments for PTSD: Practice guidelines from the International Society for Traumatic Stress Studies*. 2nd ed. New York, NY: The Guilford Press.

Forbes, David, Mark Creamer, Andrea Phelps, Richard Bryant, Alexander McFarlane, Grant J. Devilly, Lynda Matthews, Beverley Raphael, Chris Doran, Tracy Merlin, and Skye Newton. 2007. *Australian guidelines for the treatment of acute stress disorder and post-traumatic stress disorder.* Australian and New Zealand Journal of Psychiatry 41, no. 8: 637– 48. doi: 10.1080/00048670701449161 (accessed May 26, 2014).

Fullerton, Catherine Anne, Meelee Kim, Cindy Parks Thomas, D. Russell Lyman, Leslie B. Montejano, Richard H. Dougherty, Allen S. Daniels, Sushmita Shoma Ghose, and Miriam E. Delphin-Rittmon. 2013. Medication-assisted treatment with methadone: Assessing the evidence. *Psychiatric Services in Advance* (November 18): 1–12. doi: 10.1176/appi .ps.201300235 (accessed May 25, 2014).

Garfield, J. B., D. I. Lubman, and M. Yücel. 2014. Anhedonia in substance use disorders: A systematic review of its nature, course and clinical correlates. *Australian & New Zealand Journal of Psychiatry* 48, no. 1: 36–51. doi: 10.1177/0004867413508455 (accessed May 26, 2014).

Goodman, Lee-Anne. 2014. Study finds "housing first" strategy saves money, keeps people off the street. *CTV News.* April 7. http://www.ctvnews.ca/canada/study-finds-housing-first-strategy-saves-money-keeps-people-off-street-1.1765133 (accessed May 26, 2014).

Gore, T. Allen. 2014. Posttraumatic stress disorder treatment and management. *Medscape.* January 27. http://emedicine.medscape .com/article/288154-treatment (accessed May 26, 2014).

Gossop, Michael. 2005. *Drug misuse treatment and reductions in crime: Findings from the National Treatment Outcome Research Study (NTORS)* (Research Briefing 8). http://www.addictionservicesguide.com/articles /NTORS.PDF (accessed May 26, 2014).

Gossop, Michael, John Marsden, and Duncan Stewart. 2001. *NTORS after five years: Changes in substance use, health and criminal behaviour during the five years after intake* (the National Treatment Outcome Research Study). London, UK: National Addiction Centre. http://www.addictiontoday .org/addictiontoday/files/ntors_5.pdf (accessed May 25, 2014).

Graham, A. W., T. K. Schultz, M. Mayo-Smith, R. K. Ries, and B. B. Wilford, eds. 2003. *Principles of addiction medicine.* 3rd ed. Chevy Chase, MD: American Society of Addiction Medicine.

Grelotti, David J., Gen Kanayama, and Harrison G. Pope. 2010. Remission of persistent methamphetamine-induced psychosis after electroconvulsive therapy: Presentation of a case and review of the literature. *American Journal of Psychiatry* 167, no. 1: 17–23. doi: 10.1176/appi.ajp.2009.08111695 (accessed May 26, 2014).

Greydanus, Donald E., Elizabeth K. Hawver, Megan M. Greydanus, and Joav Merrick. 2013. Marijuana: Current concepts. *Frontiers in Public Health* 1: PMC3859982. doi: 10.3389/fpubh.2013.00042 (accessed May 26, 2014).

Gulliver, Suzy Bird, Barbara W. Kamholz, and Amy W. Helstrom. 2006. Smoking cessation and alcohol abstinence: What do the data tell us? *Alcohol Research & Health* 29, no. 3: 208–12. http://pubs.niaaa.nih.gov/publications/arh293/208-212.pdf (accessed May 26, 2014).

Hamblen, Jessica L., Paula Schnurr, Anna Rosenberg, and Afsoon Eftekhari. 2009. A guide to the literature on psychotherapy for PTSD. *Psychiatric Annals* 39, no. 6. doi: 10.3928/00485713-20090515-02 (accessed May 26, 2014).

Hardesty, Cameron. 2014. *5 things to know about opioid overdoses* (posted February 11). Washington, DC: The White House, Office of National Drug Control Policy. http://www.whitehouse.gov/blog/2014/02/11/5-things-know-about-opioid-overdoses (accessed May 25, 2014).

Hare, Robert D. 1991. *The Hare psychopathy checklist–revised.* North Tonawanda, NY, USA: Multi-Health Systems.

———. 2003. *Manual for the revised psychopathy checklist.* 2nd ed. Toronto, Canada: Multi-Health Systems.

Hartz, S. M., C. N. Pato, H. Medeiros, P. Cavazos-Rehg, J. L. Sobell, J. A. Knowles, and L. J. Bierut. 2014. Comorbidity of severe psychotic disorders with measures of substance abuse. *JAMA Psychiatry* 71, no. 3: 248–54. doi: 10.1001/jamapsychiatry.2013.3726 (accessed May 25, 2014).

Health Canada. 2002. *Best practices: Concurrent mental health and substance use disorders.* http://www.hc-sc.gc.ca/hc-ps/alt_formats/hecs-sesc/pdf/pubs/adp-apd/bp_disorder-mp_concomitants/bp_concurrent_mental_health-eng.pdf (accessed May 26, 2014).

———. 2013. *Information for health care professionals: Cannabis (marihuana, marijuana) and the cannabinoids.* http://www.hc-sc.gc.ca/dhp-mps/alt_formats/pdf/marihuana/med/infoprof-eng.pdf (accessed May 26, 2014).

———. 2014. *Medical use of marijuana.* http://www.hc-sc.gc.ca/dhp-mps/marihuana/index-eng.php (accessed June 30, 2014).

Health Canada's new rules to take effect April 1 prohibit medical pot users from growing at home. 2014. *CBC News.* March 21. http://www.cbc.ca/news/canada/british-columbia/medical-marijuana-users-can-grow-at-home-for-now-1.2581742 (accessed June 30, 2014).

Hudson, James I., Eva Hiripi, Harrison G. Pope, Jr., and R Ronald C. Kessler. 2007. The prevalence and correlates of eating disorders in the national comorbidity survey replication. *Biological Psychiatry* 61, no. 3: 348–58.

Huebner, Robert B., with Lori Wolfgang Kantor. 2011. Advances in alcoholism treatment. *Alcohol Research & Health* 33, no. 4: 295–9. http://pubs.niaaa.nih.gov/publications/arh334/295-299.pdf (accessed May 25, 2014).

Humphreys, K. L., T. Eng, and S. S. Lee. 2013. Stimulant medication and substance use outcomes: A meta-analysis. *JAMA Psychiatry* 70, no. 7: 740–9. doi: 10.1001/jamapsychiatry.2013.1273 (accessed May 25, 2014).

Institute of Medicine, Committee on Treatment of Posttraumatic Stress Disorder. 2008. *Treatment of posttraumatic stress disorder: An assessment of the evidence.* Washington, DC: The National Academies Press.

Kafka, Martin P. 2010. Hypersexual disorder: A proposed diagnosis for DSM-V. *Archives of Sexual Behavior*, no. 39: 377–400. doi: 10.1007/s10508-009-9574-7 (accessed May 26, 2014).

Kamal, R. M., S. van Iwaarden, B. A. Dijkstra, and C. A. de Jong. 2014. Decision rules for GHB (gamma-hydroxybutyric acid) detoxification: A vignette study. Drug and Alcohol Dependence 135 (February 1): 146– 51. doi: 10.1016/j.drugalcdep.2013.12.003

Lazo, Mariana, and Jeanne Clark. 2011. Liver function. http://www .hopkinsguides.com/hopkins/ub/view/Johns_Hopkins_Diabetes_Guid e/547086/all/Liver_function (accessed June 21, 2014).

Lecomte, Tania, Kim T. Mueser, William MacEwan, Allen E. Thornton, Tari Buchanan, Vanessa Bouchard, Elliot Goldner, Johann Brink, Donna Lang, Shimi Kang, Alasdair M. Barr, and William G. Honer. 2013. Predictors of persistent psychotic symptoms in persons with methamphetamine abuse receiving psychiatric treatment. *The Journal of Nervous and Mental Disease* 201, no. 12: 1085–9. http://journals.lww.com/jonmd/_layouts/oaks .journals.mobile/list.aspx?yearId=2013&issueId=12000&key=prev&curr entPageIndex=1&action=next (accessed May 26, 2014).

Marlatt, G. Alan, and Dennis Michael Donovan. 2005. *Relapse prevention: Maintenance strategies in the treatment of addictive behaviours*. 2nd ed. New York, NY: The Guilford Press. First published 1985.

Marlatt, G. Alan, Mary E. Larimer, and Katie Witkiewitz, eds. 2012. *Harm reduction: Pragmatic strategies for managing high-risk behaviors*. 2nd ed. New York, NY: Guilford Press.

Maté, Gabor. 2009. *In the realm of hungry ghosts: Close encounters with addiction*. Toronto, Canada: Vintage Canada.

McCarty, Dennis, Lisa Braude, D. Russell Lyman, Richard H. Dougherty, Allen S. Daniels, Sushmita Shoma Ghose, and Miriam E. Delphin-Rittmon. 2014. Substance abuse intensive outpatient programs: Assessing the evidence. *Psychiatric Services* 65, no. 6 (June). doi: 10.1176/appi.ps .201300249 (accessed July 8, 2014).

Mee-Lee, David. 2001. *ASAM PPC-2R: ASAM patient placement criteria for the treatment of substance-related disorders*. Chevy Chase, MD: American Society of Addiction Medicine (ASAM).

————. 2013. *The ASAM criteria: Treatment criteria for addictive, substance-related, and co-occurring conditions.* Chevy Chase, MD: American Society of Addiction Medicine (ASAM).

Miller, William R. 1995. *Motivational enhancement therapy manual: A clinical research guide for therapists treating individuals with alcohol abuse and dependence* (NIH Publication No. 94-3723). Rockville, MD: U.S. Department of Health and Human Services, Public Health Service, National Institutes of Health, National Institute on Alcohol Abuse and Alcoholism.

Miller, William R., and Rollnick, Stephen. 2002. *Motivational interviewing: Preparing people for change.* New York, NY: Guilford Press.

Mills, K., S. Back, K. Brady, A. Baker, M. Teesson, S. Hopwood, and C. Sannibale. 2012. *Concurrent treatment of PTSD and substance use disorders using prolonged exposure (COPE): A treatment manual* (Tech Report No. 322). Sydney, Australia: National Drug and Alcohol Research Centre (NDARC).

Najavits, Lisa M. 2002. *Seeking safety: A treatment manual for PTSD and substance abuse.* New York, NY: Guilford Press.

Narcotics Anonymous. 1988. *Narcotics Anonymous.* 5th ed. Chatsworth, CA: Narcotics Anonymous World Services. http://www.scnapi.org /downloads/NA_BASIC_TEXT_5th_edition.pdf (accessed May 26, 2014).

National Collaborating Centre for Mental Health. 2005. *Post-traumatic stress disorder (PTSD): The management of PTSD in adults and children in primary and secondary care* (Clinical Guideline 26). London, UK: National Institute for Clinical Excellence (NICE). March. http://www.nice.org.uk /nicemedia/pdf/CG026NICEguideline.pdf (accessed May 26, 2014).

National Institute on Alcohol Abuse and Alcoholism. n.d. *Helping patients who drink too much: A clinician's guide.* http://www.niaaa.nih.gov/guide (accessed May 26, 2014).

————. 2010. *Exploring treatment options for alcohol use disorders* (Alcohol Alert No. 81). http://pubs.niaaa.nih.gov/publications/AA81/AA81.htm (accessed June 21, 2014).

————. 2012. Update on the genetics of alcoholism. Alcohol *Research: Current Reviews* 34, no. 3. http://pubs.niaaa.nih.gov/publications/arcr343/toc34_3.htm (accessed May 26, 2014).

National Institute on Drug Abuse. n.d. *What treatments are effective for cocaine abusers?* (National Institute on Drug Abuse Research Report Series). https://www.drugabuse.gov/publications/research-reports/cocaine/what-treatments-are-effective-cocaine-abusers (accessed May 26, 2014).

————. 2012. *DrugFacts: Cigarettes and other tobacco products.* http://www.drugabuse.gov/publications/drugfacts/cigarettes-other-tobacco-products (accessed June 19, 2014).

————. 2013. *Research programs.* http://www.drugabuse.gov/about-nida/organization/divisions/division-pharmacotherapies-medical-consequences-drug-abuse-dpmcda/research-programs (accessed July 4, 2014).

————. 2014. *Tobacco/nicotine: Brief description.* http://www.drugabuse.gov/drugs-abuse/tobacco-nicotine (accessed May 26, 2014).

Nielsen, David A., Amol Utrankar, Jennifer A. Reyes, Daniel D. Simons, and Thomas R. Kosten. 2012. Epigenetics of drug abuse: Predisposition or response. *Pharmacogenomics* 13, no. 10: 1149–1160. doi: 10.2217/pgs.12.94 (accessed May 26, 2014).

Nunes, Edward V., and Frances R. Levin. 2008. Treatment of co-occurring depression and substance dependence: Using meta-analysis to guide clinical recommendations. *Psychiatric Annals* 38, no. 11: nihpa128505. http://www.ncbi.nlm.nih.gov/pmc/articles/PMC2722074/ (accessed May 26, 2014).

O'Donnell, Amy, Peter Anderson, Dorothy Newbury-Birch, Bernd Schulte, Christiane Schmidt, Jens Reimer, and Eileen Kaner. 2014. The impact of brief alcohol interventions in primary healthcare: A systematic review of reviews. *Alcohol and Alcoholism* 49, no. 1: 66–78. doi: 10.1093/alcalc/agt170 (accessed May 26, 2014).

Opioid overdose in BC: Fentanyl on the rise. 2013. *Toward the Heart*, no. 5 (September). http://towardtheheart.com/ezine/5/opioid-overdose-in-bc-fentanyl-on-the-rise (accessed May 26, 2014).

Opium throughout history. 2014. *PBS Frontline*. http://www.pbs.org/wgbh/pages/frontline/shows/heroin/etc/history.html (accessed July 5, 2014).

Ostacher, Michael. 2011. Bipolar and substance use disorder comorbidity: Diagnostic and treatment considerations. *Focus: The Journal of Lifelong Learning in Psychiatry* 9, no. 4 (Fall): 428–34. http://psychiatryonline.org/data/Journals/FOCUS/4393/foc00411000428.pdf_(accessed May 25, 2014).

Paulozzi, Leonard, Grant Baldwin, Gary Franklin, R. Gil Kerlikowske, Christopher M. Jones, Neelam Ghiya, and Tanja Popovic. 2012. CDC grand rounds: Prescription drug overdoses: A U.S. Epidemic. *JAMA* 307, no. 8: 774–6.

Pedersen, Traci. 2013. No link found between ADHD drugs, future substance abuse. *PsychCentral.com*. http://psychcentral.com/news/2013/06/02/no-link-found-between-adhd-drugs-future-substance-abuse/55502.html (accessed May 26, 2014).

Potts, Donald A., and John S. Daniels. Where there is smoke there must be ire! Nicotine addiction treatment: A review. 2014. *Missouri Medicine* 111, no. 1: 80–4. http://www.ncbi.nlm.nih.gov/pubmed/24645304 (accessed May 26, 2014).

Proal, Ashley C., Jerry Fleming, Juan A. Galvez-Buccollini, and Lynn E. Delisi. 2014. A controlled family study of cannabis users with and without psychosis. *Schizophrenia Research* 152, no. 1: 283–8. doi: http://dx.doi.org/10.1016/j.schres.2013.11.014 (accessed May 26, 2014).

Problem drinking. 2013. *bcguidelines.ca*. http://www.bcguidelines.ca /pdf/problem_drinking.pdf (accessed June 21, 2014).

Prochaska, James, and DiClemente, Carlo C. *The transtheoretical approach: Crossing the traditional boundaries of therapy*. Melbourne, FL: Krieger.

Public Health Agency of Canada. 2006. *The human face of mental health and mental illness in Canada 2006*. http://www.phac-aspc.gc.ca/publicat /human-humain06/pdf/human_face_e.pdf (accessed May 26, 2014).

Rehm, Ju, D. Baliunas, S. Brochu, B. Fischer, W. Gnam, J. Patra, S. Popova, A. Sarnocinska-Hart, and B. Taylor. 2006. *The costs of substance abuse in Canada 2002: Highlights*. http://www.ccsa.ca/Resource%20Library/ccsa-011332-2006.pdf (accessed May 26, 2014).

Reif, Sharon, Preethy George, Lisa Braude, Richard H. Dougherty, Allen S. Daniels, Sushmita Shoma Ghose, and Miriam E. Delphin-Rittmon. 2014. Residential treatment for individuals with substance use disorders: Assessing the evidence. *Psychiatric Services* 65, no. 3 (March). doi: 10.1176/appi.ps.201300242 (accessed July 8, 2014).

Richter, K. P., H. K. Ahluwalia, M. C. Mosier, J. Nazir, and J. S. Ahluwalia. 2002. A population-based study of cigarette smoking among illicit drug users in the united states. Addiction 97, no. 7 (July): 861–9.

Ries, Richard K., David A. Fiellin, Shannon C. Miller, and Richard Saitz. 2014. *The ASAM principles of addiction medicine*. 5th ed. Philadelphia, PA: Lippincott Williams & Wilkins.

Robins, Lee N. 1993. Vietnam veterans' rapid recovery from heroin addiction: A fluke or normal expectation? *Addiction* 88: 1041–54. http://www.rkp.wustl.edu/VESlit/RobinsAddiction1993.pdf (accessed May 26, 2014).

Robinson, Shannon. 2014. Medication for alcohol use disorder: Which agents work best? *Current Psychiatry* 13, no. 1 (January): 22–9. http://www.currentpsychiatry.com/articles/evidence-based-reviews/article/medication-for-alcohol-use-disorder-which-agents-work-best/e7f912b33d462a812cb29c8718cc852a.html (accessed May 26, 2014).

Rösner, S., A. Hackl-Herrwerth, S. Leucht, P. Lehert, S. Vecchi, and M. Soyka. 2011. Acamprosate for alcohol dependent patients. *Cochrane Summaries* (February 16). http://summaries.cochrane.org/CD004332/acamprosate-for-alcohol-dependent-patients (accessed May 25, 2014).

Sachdeva, Ankur, Mina Chandra, and Smita N. Deshpande. 2014. A comparative study of fixed tapering dose regimen versus symptom-triggered regimen of lorazepam for alcohol detoxification. *Alcohol and Alcoholism* 49, no. 3: 287–91. https://www.readbyqxmd.com/read/24407777/a-comparative-study-of-fixed-tapering-dose-regimen-versus-symptom-triggered-regimen-of-lorazepam-for-alcohol-detoxification (accessed May 26, 2014).

Salvadore, Giacomo, and Jaskaran B. Singh. 2013. Ketamine as a fast acting antidepressant: Current knowledge and open questions. *CNS Neuroscience & Therapeutics* 19, no. 6: 428–36. doi: 10.1111/cns.12103 (accessed May 26, 2014).

SMART Recovery®. 2014. *Smart Recovery: Self-management for addiction recovery*. http://www.smartrecovery.org/ (accessed May 26, 2014).

Smith, Ryan. 2014. Canada: Alberta arbitrators strike oil company's random alcohol and drug testing policy. *Mondaq.com*. April 3. http://www.mondaq.com/canada/x/304460/employee+rights+labour+relations/Alberta+Arbitrators+Strike+Oil+Companys+Random+Alcohol+And+Drug+Testing+Policy (accessed July 4, 2014).

Smyth, Bobby, Joe Barry, Alison Lane, Mary Cotter, Mary O'Neill, Caroline Quinn, and Eamon Keenan. 2005. In-patient treatment of opiate dependence: Medium-term follow-up outcomes. *The British Journal of Psychiatry* 187: 360–5. doi: 10.1192/bjp.187.4.360.

Sommer, Barbara R., Erica L. Mitchell, and Tonita E. Wroolie. 2013. Topiramate: Effects on cognition in patients with epilepsy, migraine headache and obesity. Therapeutic Advances in Neurological Disorders 6, no. 4: 211–27. doi: 10.1177/1756285613481257 (accessed July 4, 2014).

Stopping heroin use without treatment. n.d. *RecoveryStories*. http://www.recoverystories.info/stopping-heroin-use-without-treatment (accessed July 4, 2014).

Substance Abuse and Mental Health Services Administration (SAMHSA). n.d. *Screening tools.* http://www.integration.samhsa.gov/clinical-practice/screening-tools#drugs (accessed July 6, 2014).

————. 2008. *Substance abuse treatment for persons with co-occurring disorders: A treatment improvement protocol TIP 42* (SMA 13-3992). http://store.samhsa.gov/product/TIP-42-Substance-Abuse-Treatment-for-Persons-With-Co-Occurring-Disorders/SMA13-3992 (accessed May 25, 2014).

————. 2014. *SAMHSA issues advisory to treatment community on the danger of heroin contaminated with fentanyl and what can be done to save lives.* http://www.samhsa.gov/newsroom/advisories/1402075426.aspx (accessed May 26, 2014).

Supreme Court of Canada. 2013. *Communications, Energy and Paperworkers Union of Canada, Local 30 v. Irving Pulp & Paper, Ltd., 2013 SCC 34, [2013] 2 S.C.R. 458.* https://www.canlii.org/en/ca/scc/doc/2013/2013scc34/2013scc34.pdf (accessed July 4, 2014)

Synthetic cannabinoids. 2013. Call US ... The Official Newsletter of the California Poison Control System 11, no. 1 (Spring). http://www.calpoison.org/hcp/2013/callusvol11no1.htm (accessed July 4, 2014).

Szalavitz, Maia. 2012. Hazelden introduces antiaddiction medications into recovery for first time. Time. November 5. http://healthland.time.com/2012/11/05/hazelden-introduces-antiaddiction-medications-in-recovery-for-first-time/ (accessed May 25, 2014).

————. 2013. ADHD medication in childhood does not increase addiction risk. *Time.* May 30. http://healthland.time.com/2013/05/30/adhd-medication-in-childhood-does-not-increase-addiction-risk/ (accessed May 26, 2014).

Thompson, Pamela J., S. A. Baxendale, J. S. Duncan, and J. W. Sander. 2000. Effects of topiramate on cognitive function. *Journal of Neurology, Neurosurgery & Psychiatry* 69, no. 5: 636– 41. doi: 10.1136/jnnp.69.5.636 (accessed July 4, 2014).

Trimpey, Jack. 1996. Rational recovery: The new cure for substance addiction. New York, NY: Gallery Books.

United Nations Office on Drugs and Crime (UNODC). 2014. *Details for synthetic cannabinoids.* https://www.unodc.org/LSS/SubstanceGroup/Details/ae45ce06-6d33-4f5f-916a-e873f07bde02 (accessed May 25, 2014).

Vaillant, George E. 2003. Natural history of addiction and pathways to recovery. In *Principles of addiction medicine,* ed. A. W. Graham, T. K. Schultz, M. Mayo-Smith, Richard K. Ries, and B. B. Wilford, 3–16. 3rd ed. Chevy Chase, MD: American Society of Addiction Medicine.

Van Emmerik-van Oortmerssen, Katelijne, Geurt Van de Glind, Wim Van den Brink, Filip Smit, Cleo L. Crunelle, Marije Swets, and Robert A. Schoevers. 2012. Prevalence of attention-deficit hyperactivity disorder in substance use disorder patients: A meta-analysis and meta-regression analysis. *Drug and Alcohol Dependence* 122, no. 1-2: 11–9. http://dare.uva.nl/document/498780 (accessed May 26, 2014).

Volkow, Nora D., Ruben D. Baler, Wilson M. Compton, and Susan R. B. Weiss. 2014. Adverse health effects of marijuana use. *New England Journal of Medicine* 370, no. June 5: 2219–27. doi: 10.1056/NEJMra1402309 (accessed June 30, 2014).

Volkow, Nora D., Thomas R. Frieden, Pamela S. Hyde, and Stephen S. Cha. 2014. Medication-assisted therapies: Tackling the opioid-overdose epidemic. New England Journal of Medicine 370, no. 22: 2063–6. doi: 10.1056/NEJMp1402780.

Volkow, Nora D., Gene-Jack Wang, Dardo Tomasi, and Ruben D. Baler. 2013. The addictive dimensionality of obesity. *Biological Psychiatry* 73, no. 9: 811–8. doi: http://dx.doi.org/10.1016/j.biopsych.2012.12.020 (accessed May 26, 2014).

WebMD. 2014. ADHD and substance abuse. http://www.webmd.com/add-adhd/guide/adhd-and-substance-abuse-is-there-a-link (accessed May 26, 2014).

White, William L. 2012. *Recovery/remission from substance use disorders* (An analysis of reported outcomes in 415 scientific reports, 1868–2011). http://www.naadac.org/assets/1959/whitewl2012_recoveryremission_from_substance_abuse_disorders.pdf (accessed June 21, 2014).

World Health Organization. 2012. *Management of substance abuse: Alcohol.* http://www.who.int/substance_abuse/facts/alcohol/en/ (accessed July 4, 2014).

Made in the USA
Charleston, SC
09 November 2015